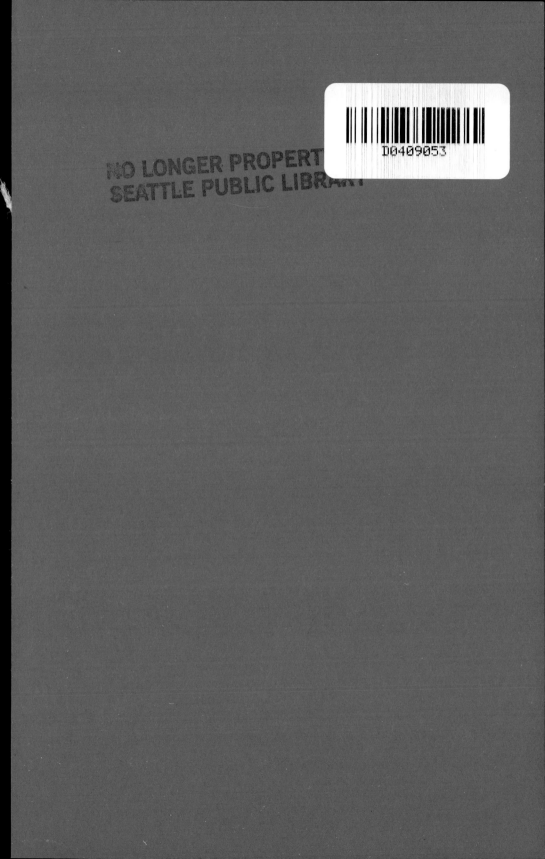

D0409053

THE FEARS OF THE RICH, THE NEEDS OF THE POOR

THE FEARS OF THE RICH, THE NEEDS OF THE POOR

My Years at the CDC

WILLIAM H. FOEGE

Johns Hopkins University Press | *Baltimore*

Johns Hopkins University Press
2715 North Charles Street
Baltimore, Maryland 21218-4363
www.press.jhu.edu

Library of Congress Cataloging-in-Publication Data

Names: Foege, William H., 1936– author.
Title: The fears of the rich, The needs of the poor : my years at the CDC / William H.
    Foege.
Description: Baltimore : Johns Hopkins University Press, [2018] | Includes
    bibliographical references and index.
Identifiers: LCCN 2017035213| ISBN 9781421425290 (hardcover : alk. paper) |
    ISBN 1421425297 (hardcover : alk. paper) | ISBN 9781421425306 (electronic) |
    ISBN 1421425300 (electronic)
Subjects: | MESH: Foege, William H., 1936– | Centers for Disease Control and
    Prevention (US) | Public Health Administration | Public Health Practice |
    Communicable Disease Control | United States Government Agencies |
    United States | Personal Narratives
Classification: LCC RA425 | NLM WA 540 AA1 | DDC 362.1—dc23
    LC record available at https://lccn.loc.gov/2017035213

A catalog record for this book is available from the British Library.

*Special discounts are available for bulk purchases of this book. For more information, please contact
Special Sales at 410-516-6936 or specialsales@press.jhu.edu.*

Johns Hopkins University Press uses environmentally friendly book materials, including recycled
text paper that is composed of at least 30 percent post-consumer waste, whenever possible.

For Paula, David, Michael, Robert, Max, Ella, Olyana, and Erika

CONTENTS

Preface ix

1. A Threat 1
2. Security: How Much Is Enough? 4
3. Lassa and Ebola 7
4. A Short History of the CDC 18
5. The Fears of the Rich and the Needs of the Poor 28
6. Balancing Babies and the Marketplace 43
7. Toxic Shock: Unexpected Deaths from an Improved Product 47
8. Serendipity and Unexpected Paths 51
9. The Mysterious Deaths of Veterans 58
10. An Unexpected Return to the CDC 69
11. Disaster Relief 79
12. Smallpox Claims Its Last Victims 93
13. Coming into the United States: New Americans 98
14. Organizing for Success 104
15. Vaccines: The Foundation of Public Health 126
16. Do No Harm 148
17. Global Health: Sharing Our Science 153
18. Positive Politics 162
19. Toxic Politics 170
20. Reye Syndrome: Following the Evidence 179
21. Comic Relief 187
22. Reducing the Toll of Injuries 195
23. Uncommon People 200
24. AIDS: Overwhelming Public Health 209
25. Blind Spots 225
26. On Budgets and Burglars 233

Acknowledgments 239
Appendix. Voices in My Head 241
References 253
Index 257

PREFACE

Modern public health can be traced to May 14, 1796, when Edward Jenner inoculated a young boy, James Phipps, with cowpox material taken from a sore on the hand of Sarah Nelmes, a milkmaid infected with cowpox. Jenner was trying to mimic nature. He had observed that milkmaids appeared to be protected from smallpox disease. A subsequent attempt to infect Phipps with smallpox was unsuccessful. The boy had been protected by the cowpox inoculation.

Although many references to prevention and public health are found in both biblical and other historic writings, Jenner's success marked the first time an actual tool was available to improve individual health and the health of people in the aggregate. Modern public health was now possible.

Linking public health, and specifically the Centers for Disease Control and Prevention (CDC), to Jenner's work is an acknowledgment of our debt to that event. The CDC originally focused on communicable diseases, and immunizations and vaccines continue to be the foundation of public health. But the field has been expanded in one lifetime to encompass occupational hazards, environmental problems, intentional and unintentional injuries, chronic diseases, and mental health. The mission now embraces all types of barriers to health—biological, chemical, behavioral, violent, and environmental—and recognizes positive ways to enhance quality of life.

I have been a list keeper throughout my life, keeping track of countries visited, trips taken, books read, quotations recalled, and lessons learned. Over the years, I have been intrigued by mentors I have never met, except through reading, and I have tried to divine what advice they might have had for me at different junctures in my life. Many of these influences, in one form or another, made it into this book.

This book is not a history of the CDC nor is it a history of public health or the breadth of CDC activities. It is a collection of stories. By telling these stories, I hope to illuminate the roles that, thanks to the CDC, my colleagues and I played at important moments in the history of global health and to reveal some of the lessons learned along the way.

THE FEARS OF THE RICH, THE NEEDS OF THE POOR

chapter 1

A THREAT

My assistant entered the office, handed me a letter, and said, "You had better read this before you do anything else." The writer informed me that he or she could deposit, undetected, botulinum toxin in a city water supply. This toxin is one of the most lethal agents known: a single teaspoon can kill millions of people. This was serious business. The writer provided sufficient detail to indicate he knew the subject well. He would be willing to negotiate if I would put an ad in the personals section of the *New York Times* with the message provided by the writer. I called the Federal Bureau of Investigation (FBI).

This threatening letter was one of many letters addressed to the director of the Centers for Disease Control (CDC) and received every day in the CDC front office. If left to me, it might have taken days before I would have opened it. But we had a system: my assistant, Carol Walters, opened every letter and logged them in to be sure they received attention and got answered. Carol had taken this letter from the pile and brought it to me. She was alarmed.

Botulinum toxin, an extremely toxic protein, is produced by a bacterium called *Clostridium botulinum*. The bacterium stays viable for long periods by encapsulating into a spore. It can grow only in an oxygen-deprived environment. Food poisoning, long feared in home-canned products, results from inadequate heating after jars are sealed, which allows spores to begin to grow in the canned food. The bacterium then produces a toxin, which has a devastating effect on the person eating that food. The toxin blocks the release of acetylcholine in muscles, which prevents the muscles from contracting. People die because they cannot breathe when the chest muscles become paralyzed.

We may have lost some of the fear of this toxin for two reasons. Home-canned food is less common now. Moreover, we use a diluted injectable form of botulinum toxin, or BOTOX, as a cosmetic aid that paralyzes small muscles that cause the wrinkles of aging. (When diluted, botulinum toxin's toxicity can be restricted to certain muscles.) It's easy to forget how toxic the substance can be.

The FBI questioned CDC botulism experts, out of prudence, but also to determine the letter writer's level of expertise. Some of the letter's language included recent findings, an indication that the writer was an expert in the field or at least aware of recent literature. The FBI took the threat seriously. Federal agents took the letter for analysis. As with any homicide investigation, detectives must first rule out those closest to the victim. We had to ask whether any of our experts could be involved. After our suspicions were allayed, the FBI arranged to place the classified ad as instructed by the letter writer.

A second letter followed the classified ad's publication; it contained additional details of the writer's plan and a request for a second classified ad in the *New York Times*. The FBI continued their analyses and began to focus on an area in Florida as the source of the letters. The agency had been able to determine the brand of typewriter used and had hopes of finding the writer. Another letter might provide the breakthrough the FBI needed.

But suddenly things changed. The FBI called me one morning to say that a journalist had gotten wind of the investigation and was about to file a report. The journalist would be contacting me for details, and I was urged to get the journalist to delay reporting the incident.

The reporter did call me. I begged him to wait for the FBI to have a chance to apprehend the individual. We could provide the journalist with an exclusive report at that time. He refused, the report was published, and we never heard from the letter writer again. What kept the person from carrying out the threat? How many other people have similar interests? How do we balance the need for transparency, freedom of the press, and protecting the public?

This serious episode led the CDC to develop a defensive bioterrorism strategy in the early 1980s. The program, headed by Stuart Kingma, public health advisor at the CDC, involved a review of every organism that the CDC staff felt could be used for warfare or terrorism and the development of counterterrorism steps that could be taken. Stuart Kingma was the right person for this assignment. Tall, fit, and thoughtful, he brought a Dutch attention to detail to everything he did. From hunting to building boats and telescopes to making ceramics, he researched everything and insisted on perfection. He eventually had a person in charge of every organism determined to be a potential risk, and a program was developed with the FBI so that someone would always be on call if CDC assistance were needed. Secure communications were installed, and a secure conference room was developed at the CDC.

When the defense plan was complete, I naively thought we could classify it. However, I found, to my dismay, that the CDC had no way to classify documents. As a result, this plan would have to be released if requested under the Freedom of Information Act. Our work with the FBI revealed that concerns regarding bioterrorism were shared in many parts of government. The largest body of expertise was probably in the US Department of Defense, which indicated a readiness to hear about the CDC assessment. I took a copy of the plan to my contact at the Defense Department. As he read through the plan, he looked up to ask me why it wasn't classified. I told him that the CDC lacked that authority. He then did what I had hoped for. He said, "Well, I have that authority," and he stamped it "classified."

Twenty years later, when anthrax spores were transmitted through the US mail in 2001, the CDC no longer had a bioterrorism program. Why? After being briefed on the program in the 1980s, a CDC manager concluded, "that will never happen," and dismantled the CDC biodefense program!

chapter 2

SECURITY

How Much Is Enough?

Microbes seem to get into the CDC without any trouble. But it is harder for people. As I revisited the CDC in 2011 (twenty-six years after leaving my post there) for the dedication of a museum in honor of former CDC Director David Sencer, guards required identification for me to get to the parking deck. I then needed to show a picture ID at the entrance to the building, and someone in the CDC building needed to clear me. An identification badge was issued, and airport-like security machines examined me and my briefcase. It mattered not that I was once the director of this federal agency. Without a pass and an escort, I could not enter. And that is exactly as it should be.

This visit brought back memories of why we implemented increasingly stringent security measures. It was 1977, and the CDC's open buildings were easily accessible, like a university campus or an organization that wanted to encourage use during evenings and weekends. Scientists were always returning at odd times to check on an experiment, to follow up on work, or to make phone contact with people in other time zones.

On February 18, 1977, mild upper respiratory symptoms developed in two CDC employees; they seemed to recover but then became feverish on February 23. Within days, both were hospitalized and then both died. Rocky Mountain spotted fever was the cause of their deaths. Although no break in technique or laboratory accident could be identified, it was a frightening reminder that we had to improve security.

At about the same time, we were troubled when a postal employee, attempting to deliver a package, walked into the smallpox laboratory and asked for a person by name. The CDC had led a successful effort to eradicate smallpox from West and Central Africa, had posted dozens of workers to other countries, especially to India and Bangladesh, and received specimens from around the world daily to test them for smallpox. So we worried about the chance of the CDC's being the source of virus for new outbreaks. Warnings were posted on the doors to the lab to indicate that employees were working with smallpox and that no one could enter who was not properly vaccinated. Posted warnings were sufficient for others working at the CDC, but they had to be read to be useful, and clearly they were not adequate to keep a US postal employee from his appointed rounds. Our response was to install a card-key system for all buildings. Individual cards were programmed to allow access to any building deemed necessary for that employee. While not adequate for true security (since one employee could borrow the card of another employee), it was adequate for inadvertent access to dangerous areas.

Health Risk Appraisals

My 2011 visit to the CDC also reminded me of our first use of a computerized health risk appraisal program. If an employee answered questions on his or her health history and health practices, it was possible to provide that individual with a clever incentive to improve health habits. A response might indicate that a 55-year-old employee had the health risks of a 62-year-old. However, by following the recommendations on smoking, exercising, and weight loss, the employee could again have the biological age of a 48-year-old. That is compelling.

As part of the form, people answered questions on, among other practices, the frequency of seat-belt use, drinking habits, and whether they carried a knife or gun. These data all figured into the appraisal of health risks. We could not see the results for any one person—only that person had access to that information—but we could get aggregate results.

Some years earlier at an Epidemic Intelligence Service (EIS) conference, a paper had been presented on canine rabies and its associated risks. Suddenly, Cecil Reinstein, the health officer in Grand Junction, Colorado, stood up and said, "Here is how we handle rabies in Colorado." To the astonishment of everyone, he pulled a pistol from his waistband and shot a blank into the air.

The 1977 Health Risk Appraisal results took me back to that display of a gun at the EIS conference, and for the first time, I had an indication of how common it was for CDC employees to come to work with a knife or a gun in their briefcase or on their person. In those days, it was a startlingly common practice, which may have been true for many organizations. (In reporting the results of this test at our small staff meeting, I said, "I have started being nicer to people.")

Thanks to obvious security concerns, such days are only memories at the CDC. But security issues are ever present. CDC workers are faced not only with the security of the building but also with the security of the country and, in very real ways, the security of the world. The stories are scary and frequent.

In the case of the EIS, security is part of its very mission. The EIS was created in 1951 by the legendary Alexander Langmuir because of the nation's fear of biological warfare. The intent was to develop an elite cadre of disease detectives able to diagnose and characterize outbreaks of infectious diseases that might have been deliberately initiated. Over the years, this group has provided outstanding public health assistance by investigating thousands of outbreaks of adverse health events around the world, both infectious and noninfectious problems, offering solutions and improving the knowledge of the natural history of health problems.*

*Langmuir was, as the saying goes, from central casting. Well trained, with an MD from Harvard and a master of public health degree from Johns Hopkins, he had served as an epidemiologist in the military during World War II and arrived at the CDC at the age of 39, brimming with experience and confidence. He expected much from himself and those working with him, and he got it. Outspoken, direct, sometimes fearsome, he was actually a concerned supervisor who was willing to assist his charges in any way they needed. This inspired incredible loyalty.

chapter 3

LASSA AND EBOLA

On average, the world experiences one or more new emerging communicable disease problems each year. Often they are known conditions whose cause is suddenly revealed. Legionellosis, to be discussed later, falls into this category. Other times, an organism is enhanced by some change in how we do things. Toxic shock syndrome is an old problem, for example, but a new type of tampon, introduced in the late 1970s, enhanced its incidence, causing a widespread, frightening outbreak among menstruating women. Sometimes a slight variation in an old organism provides new threats. The introduction of new influenza strains is a constant concern for the public health community, for example. And sometimes we actually identify new organisms not previously recognized. Lassa and Ebola virus infections, which suddenly arose in Africa in 1969 and 1976, were newly discovered pathogens but, undoubtedly, had been causing disease in Africa for many years. Sometimes the problem is indeed new, as with AIDS.

Lassa Fever

Nurse Lily Lyman Pinneo led a life of adventure and service—and had a very close call. Pinneo grew up in a family of medical people and missionaries. After obtaining a nursing degree from the Johns Hopkins Hospital

School for Nurses, she arrived in Nigeria a year after the end of World War II. She started a health care center in Jos, Nigeria, which soon acquired a doctor and additional nurses and became known as the Bingham Hospital.

January 1969 would be known by some as the date of release of the first Led Zeppelin album. Others would recall it as the date that Richard Nixon was inaugurated the thirty-seventh president of the United States. Pinneo would recall it as the beginning of a nightmare. That month, an American nurse, working in Lassa, a village east of Jos, became sick with fever that progressed to hemorrhagic symptoms. She was flown to Bingham Hospital, where she died within a day. One week later, a nurse at Bingham Hospital became sick with the same symptoms and died.

Nurse Pinneo had cared for both of these nurses, and now she developed symptoms. Her temperature was said to have reached 107 degrees. She was flown to Lagos and was hospitalized and cared for by Stan Foster, a CDC physician working on smallpox eradication.

It was decided that Pinneo needed to be cared for in the United States, and she was flown to New York on a commercial flight. Her area on the plane was curtained off from the rest of the cabin. Lyle Conrad, another CDC physician, cared for her on the flight.

On arrival in New York, John Frame, a physician at the Columbia-Presbyterian Hospital, drew blood samples and sent them, along with specimens from the two nurses who had died, to the Yale Arborvirus Research Unit. Pinneo was admitted to Columbia-Presbyterian Hospital, where doctors ruled out every known tropical disease.

Meanwhile, at the Yale lab, three physicians (Jordi Casals, Sonja Buckley, and Wilbur Downs) studied the samples. No one else was involved in the studies or handled the blood specimens. When Dr. Casals became ill, he assumed he had the flu. But he was persuaded to be admitted to Columbia-Presbyterian Hospital, where the staff suspected he had the same, as yet unnamed, illness as Pinneo. The staff suspicions turned out to be correct.

The hospital staff tried something radical. With no treatment available for Dr. Casals, they drew two units of blood from Pinneo and separated her plasma, which they reasoned would, with her recovery, contain the antibodies that had defeated the virus in her body. They were correct; Dr. Casals received Pinneo's antibodies and recovered.

But there was one more shock. Back at Yale, Juan Roman, a laboratory worker with no known contact with the specimens, developed hemorrhagic fever and died. Yale ceased work on the virus and sent its specimens to the CDC in Atlanta. There, the virus was ultimately isolated and characterized as a single-stranded ribonucleic acid (RNA) virus. How common was the illness? How could it be diagnosed? Was there a way to treat patients with the virus? All were unanswered questions.

Pinneo returned to her work at Bingham Hospital in 1970. She arrived with vials of her own convalescent-phase plasma antibodies to treat other patients with the disease. Her arrival came too late for staff physician Jeanette Troup, from Colorado, who had performed an autopsy on a patient who had Lassa fever. Dr. Troup had incurred a cut during the autopsy and subsequently developed Lassa fever. She died ten days before Pinneo returned with her lifesaving plasma.

Pinneo continued her work as nurse-midwife but also continued to work on Lassa fever both in Nigeria and in other West African countries. After forty years of work in Africa, she retired in the United States. She died on August 17, 2012, at age 95. The Pinneo strain of Lassa fever was named in recognition of her being the first person to have laboratory-confirmed Lassa fever.

Meanwhile, Joseph McCormick and other scientists at the CDC studied the virus, the disease it caused, and the means of transmission. They found that the disease is common in West Africa, resulting in about 5,000 deaths a year and perhaps 500,000 cases of illness. That means the fatality rate is only about 1 percent because, in most cases, it is a mild and unrecognized illness. If the illness is sufficiently severe to bring a person to the hospital, up to 20 percent will die.

Why the string of four American deaths in a single chain of transmission? It could be that the strain was unusually deadly, that the outsiders had no immunity from an earlier exposure to less lethal strains (a significant percentage of Nigerians were later shown to have antibodies to the virus), or a combination of several factors.

Dr. McCormick discovered that the *Mastomys* rat of West Africa is a reservoir for Lassa virus. This rat is widely found in the savannas and forests of West Africa, but it appears to enjoy living in human homes. In an interview (1), McCormick described his understanding of the spread of the virus:

One way is from the urine of the rodent *Mastomys natalensis*, which is the common rodent called the "multi-man" rat that you find throughout much of Africa, as a matter of fact, but especially in West Africa. This rodent tends to live in houses with humans. It will live there for long periods of time. What usually happens in West Africa is that the people wake up in the morning, they get a bit of breakfast, and then they close their houses up, leaving them dark inside, and go off to their day's activities. Of course, when they come back in the evening, it becomes dark at 6:30 p.m. or 7 p.m., and what this means for the rodent is that it sometimes has almost 24 hours of nighttime activity. During that time, the rodent will circulate through the house and deposit urine on surfaces such as the floors, the tables, and even in food if the rodent is able to get into the food and other places . . . even on beds. And we believe that people get infected most frequently when they come into contact with the deposited rodent urine on one of these surfaces, usually transmitting the virus through cuts and scratches on their hands and feet.

Another method of spread is person to person, as with the nurses at Jos.

While a vaccine is not available, work continues on vaccine development, and a treatment is now available. Ribavirin, an antiviral drug, appears effective if it is administered early and intravenously.

Ebola Hemorrhagic Disease

Other new, deadly, and frankly scary viruses continue to be discovered and understood. One is Ebola.

It was August 1976. Gerald Ford had just won the Republican presidential nomination but would lose the election to Jimmy Carter. Thousands had died in an earthquake and tidal wave in the Philippines, and thousands more had died in an earthquake in China. But none of that mattered to 44-year-old Mabalo Lokela, a teacher in Yambuku, Zaire. He was feeling lousy, and because of a high fever, he went to the local hospital.

The hospital was always overburdened, forced to treat many people on an outpatient basis for conditions that would have automatically led to hospitalization in Europe or in the United States. One of the nurses assumed Lokela had malaria and gave him a shot of quinine. She had no way of knowing that, in truth, he was the first known case in an epidemic of a previously unrecognized disease, Ebola hemorrhagic fever.

Over the years, this disease would spread fear in villages in Africa (especially in Uganda, The Congo, and Sudan), in workers exposed to outbreaks, and in countries around the world that feared an importation of the virus. How Lokela got the Ebola virus is unclear. A third of a century later, the natural history of this virus is still under investigation. Thousands of tests on animals, insects, and birds now cast suspicion on three types of fruit bats. It is believed that they can carry and spread the disease without becoming ill, thereby providing a reservoir for the virus between human outbreaks. Fruit bats may spread the virus to people directly or through animals.

What is clear is that other people in the hospital got the virus from the inadequately cleaned syringe and needle used to administer the quinine to Lokela, as well as from close personal contact with him.

Lokela was sent home, where he died. The women of his family prepared his body for the traditional funeral, a ritual that included removing blood from his body. Most of them soon also developed Ebola infections and died.

At the hospital, if there had been only one break in hygiene, it might have led to an additional case. But the actual break in hygiene was far more substantial. The hospital had only a handful of needles, and these were used over and over. The staff lacked the time and inclination for suitable sterilization between patients. Many patients, admitted for a wide spectrum of health concerns, were about to share a common problem due to contaminated needles. Previous outbreaks of the disease had probably occurred, but Lokela's was the world's first recognized outbreak of Ebola hemorrhagic fever.

When the government of Zaire realized that they were faced with a terrifying hemorrhagic disease problem, they requested help, and an international response was launched by the World Health Organization (WHO) with the help of the CDC. The team included physicians Karl Johnson from the CDC, a well-known expert in hemorrhagic fevers; Joel Breman, a veteran of the smallpox program; Joe McCormick, mentioned earlier, who had grown up in Africa and worked with highly dangerous viruses; and Peter Piot, who would later head up the United Nations AIDS (acquired immunodeficiency syndrome) program. Later, Mike White, an epidemiologist from CDC, would join the team.

These were experienced scientists, but the risks involved in such an outbreak are sobering. Investigators do not know what the agent is, and they don't know whether it is a newly recognized virus. (In this case, it turned out to be a newly recognized virus and one of the most lethal known.) If the agent is new, scientists don't know anything about its method of spread, lethality, infectiousness, incubation period, or susceptibility to usual containment measures. They don't know whether it is airborne and, if so, how far it can be transmitted through the air. Will it go meters or hundreds of meters? They don't know whether apparently healthy people can spread the agent to others. Everything is cause for worry. In addition, scientists in such situations need to work in special quarantine suits that make the tropical heat even more unbearable. One can stay only an hour or less in such a suit before seeking relief, which raised another concern: how do you avoid contamination from the outside of the suit as you remove it?

On the flight from Geneva, Switzerland, to Kinshasa, Democratic Republic of the Congo, Breman and Piot met one of the most important people of the entire response operation. William Close, an American physician and father of actress Glenn Close, was on his way to the United States on home leave when he heard of the outbreak and immediately returned to Zaire. Raised in France and educated in England and the United States, Dr. Close was a pilot during World War II and attended medical school at Columbia University. In Kinshasa, he ran the large Mama Yemo Hospital and was the personal physician for President Mobutu Sese Seko. Dr. Close became a crucial link in the outbreak investigation, procuring refrigerators, supplies, permits, and even the president's personal aircraft to provide transportation for the investigation team members and the supplies they required.

The WHO/CDC team found chaos and fear. And they had an overwhelming to-do list. They had to find the people with the disease and provide them with quarantine, food, and shelter to make sure they were no threat to others. They had to locate the dead to find whether next of kin were sick. They had to do a house-to-house survey of the town and the surrounding areas. They had to characterize the outbreak. Who was the index case-patient? What chains of infection extended from that case? Who were now at risk? The scientists had to get specimens for lab analysis, attempt to isolate an organism, and then look for antibodies to that organism in sick and in well people. They had to identify survivors and determine why they had survived. They also had to figure out the natural history of this organism. Was it usually confined to an animal species with occasional infections of humans? Would it become a permanent and ongoing human disease? Were insects or animals involved as vectors?

And always, the scientists were dealing with unrelenting heat and rain, suffocating humidity, difficulty sleeping, and the unsettling presence of insects and rodents. Amid all of this, they had to find a place to stay and an area for washing themselves and their potentially contaminated clothes without endangering others. They had to arrange for food, transportation, and communications in Yambuku and surrounding villages, where they were strangers and did not speak the local Ngbandi language. There is nothing easy about this kind of investigation. It sounds exciting and glamorous only to those who have never been in this situation.

The team, with the help of Dr. Close, managed to import protective equipment for investigators and clinicians who cared for patients. They also imported medical supplies, sterilization equipment, and necessities for quarantining patients. To quarantine a patient so he or she cannot transmit the virus requires providing everything the patient needs. This includes food, water, medicines, clothing, blankets, and pillows. Otherwise, the patient will find a way out or loved ones will find a way in. A complication is the possibility of feverish patients', unaware of what they are doing, trying to break out of a strange and terrifying environment.

The team determined that this was a devastating outbreak with unbelievably high mortality rates. They would eventually identify 318 cases, 280 fatal. The area was seized by understandable panic. When 11 of the medical staff at the hospital died, even the hospital was forced to close down. Ironically, the inability to continue staffing the hospital was important to halting the outbreak because contaminated needles and syringes were an important vehicle of transmission. Yambuku and surrounding villages were considered quarantined and visits from other areas were discouraged. President Mobutu flew to France to escape the outbreak.

The best guess initially was that the virus might be Marburg or a variation of that virus. Marburg virus was first recognized in the 1960s, in Germany, after humans were exposed to tissues of infected African green monkeys from Uganda. Of the 31 persons infected, 7 died of hemorrhagic fever.

When it was determined this was a virus never previously isolated, the investigators had the privilege of naming it. To name the virus after the village, as had been done with Lassa fever, could lead to long-term bias against the people of the village. It was decided to name it after the Ebola River, not the closest river but close enough to identify an area.

The isolation of cases and close surveillance of contacts finally brought the outbreak to an end. But the team left, after trapping many animals and insects, without understanding the natural hosts of the virus or what caused its crossover to humans.

And then it was found that an earlier outbreak had been in process but not initially recognized as a new disease. Two months before the first case in Yambuku, a storekeeper in Nzara township in Sudan had become ill with fever, headache, and chest pain. He was admitted to the hospital on June 20 and died on July 6, 1976. A brother also developed symptoms but recovered.

Again, the WHO organized an international response. The team had members from France, Germany, the United Kingdom, and the United States, including Dr. Don Francis, who had distinguished himself in the Smallpox Eradication Program; CDC performed many of the laboratory tests. Again, the team had to contend with all of the problems inherent in the Zaire investigation with little knowledge of the things being learned in Zaire.

These scientists eventually discovered 284 cases of Ebola hemorrhagic fever, about half fatal. It was later determined that the Ebola strain in Sudan was slightly different from the strain in Zaire.

Similar to the Zaire outbreak in many ways, the Sudan outbreak was magnified by both direct contact with patients and the amplifying potential of a hospital. The initial outbreak was concentrated in Nzara but then spread to Maridi, 75 miles away, where 213 of the 284 cases appeared.

This was the beginning of the ongoing odyssey with the Ebola virus. There have been dozens of outbreaks and hundreds of deaths recognized since that time. Each one brings fear and uncertainty, heroism from clinicians and families, and mystery for responders.

On at least five occasions the outbreaks have involved more than 100 persons. In 2014, an outbreak occurred in Guinea, a first for that area, but then spread to Liberia, Sierra Leone, Nigeria, and Senegal. By far the largest outbreak of Ebola recorded, it led to global concern. On August 2, 2014, the first person with Ebola infection was moved to the United States and admitted to Emory University in Atlanta for intensive care. Others were to follow.

Each outbreak has been tragic. But until the 2014 outbreak, not one outbreak has bothered me as much as the outbreak in Gulu, Uganda, in 2000. On October 7, 2000, the medical director of St. Mary's Hospital, Dr. Matthew Lukwiya was on leave to attend a course in public health. He received an urgent request to return to the hospital because of a mysterious illness that had killed two student nurses. He arrived back at the hospital that night, just as a third nurse died. He evaluated the evidence presented and spent the night reading reports from the CDC and the WHO. By morning, he concluded the hospital was dealing with Ebola virus, and he set up a model response to the outbreak.

Dr. Lukwiya was an uncommonly gifted man. His father had drowned when Matthew was 12. His mother was a petty trader, and that was his expected future. He was already learning how to smuggle goods from Sudan to be sold in markets in Uganda. But he was a gifted student, and he led his class in grade school and secondary school. There are many gifted children in Africa, but few have the opportunity to develop those gifts because of scarce resources or the lack of a system for recognizing their gifts. Matthew was different and fortunate. Teachers recognized his abilities and urged him to continue school. He received scholarships that allowed him to go beyond secondary school to the university and, then, with more help from others, he was able to attend medical school. He became an intern at St. Mary's Hospital. Within three months, the founders of the hospital were so impressed with him that they decided they had found its next medical direc-

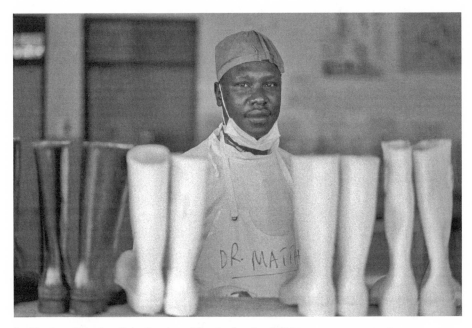

Dr. Matthew Lukwiya, Gulu, Northern Nigeria, October 2000. Photo by Seamus Murphy, courtesy of Panos Pictures

tor. He was sponsored for a pediatric degree at Liverpool with the expectation that he would return to St. Mary's Hospital to take up the medical director position.

Dr. Lukwiya turned down offers to remain in Liverpool and returned, as planned, to lead St. Mary's to new heights. His ambition to understand all aspects of medicine had led to the training sabbatical for a public health degree. In the midst of that training in 2000, he was called back to determine the cause of the deaths and to lead the effort to stop the outbreak.

He set up an isolation ward and developed such an efficient response that when the WHO team arrived, they found they had little to suggest. But this is not a forgiving virus. Any break in protocol can place one at risk.

After six weeks of exhausting work, Dr. Lukwiya made his one mistake. He was awakened from a sound sleep on November 20 because one patient, close to death and probably no longer aware of what he was doing, got up, pulled out his tubes, and walked out of the ward. Dr. Lukwiya, on awakening, put on all of his protective clothing, including two pairs of gloves. But in his haste to respond to a man who was exposing others to this deadly virus, he forgot his goggles and face shield. He quickly worked to guide the man back to his isolation ward. It was a short exposure and the path of the virus is unknown, but somehow the virus managed to make it from the patient to Dr. Lukwiya.

The patient died within the hour. Six days later Dr. Lukwiya developed "the flu," and he and the nurse diagnosed malaria. But they feared worse. Dr. Pierre Rollin, from the CDC, took blood for testing. He diagnosed Ebola, and Dr. Lukwiya entered the isolation ward that he had designed. I can only imagine what a depressing moment that must have been, when the person who knew most about the virus and its means of spread, suddenly realized that something had gone wrong in all of the precautions that had been taken. He appeared to be improving and then hemorrhaged into his lungs and died on December 5, 2000. It was a tragedy for everyone—his family, the hospital, his future patients, the country, and the world. Superior intelligence was no match for this diabolical virus.

As I write this, the world is in the throes of an outbreak of Ebola, unlike any seen before. The outbreak was the first in West Africa. For months, as Dr. Thomas Frieden, then director of CDC, told *Time* magazine (2), the WHO did not want the help of the CDC. Within months, it was clear the outbreak exceeded the capacity of the WHO and help materialized from the CDC and many other sources. Ebola spread rapidly and soon included urban areas. Three countries—Liberia, Sierra Leone, and Guinea—bore the brunt of the outbreak. Nigeria, Senegal, and Mali also had cases but controlled the outbreak quite rapidly.

By December 2014, there were still hundreds of new cases a day in West Africa, and even the United States had cases and two deaths.

Thirty-six years after the first outbreak, we do not want to learn so many new lessons. If we thought this was chaotic in rural areas, it was absolute bedlam in urban areas. The virus spread in treatment facilities, at home, and especially during the traditional burial practices, in which bodies are washed, there is close contact, and often times many loved ones touch the body.

Care of the sick was needed. Finally, with the assistance of military units from the United States and other countries, facilities began to meet the need. But the epicenter continued to shift, and therefore facilities were not always available.

The lessons of the first outbreaks, to isolate cases and follow contacts closely, looking especially for fever, paid off in the recent West African outbreak, when Ebola was imported to Lagos, Nigeria. This could have been an urban disaster but was quickly contained by Nigerian epidemiologists trained by the CDC. These epidemiologists swung into action and made hundreds of home visits, following contacts, looking for fever and signs of illness. The outbreak in Lagos was quickly contained.

We now know the following steps are also critical in Ebola outbreaks: global coordination of facilities for care and isolation; clinical care of the sick; point-of-service diagnostic abilities to avoid moving blood specimens out of the patient area and to get rapid results; assistance in burying those who die; logistic support for everything from obtaining supplies to providing transportation of patients, food, and other assistance; and superb surveillance, analysis, and communication with all who need information.

There were lessons beyond the scientific findings. Public health infectious disease outbreaks can destroy local economies and have worldwide implications. The constant drumbeat of nations trying to reduce the WHO budget was successful in keeping down that organization's growth—and it was absolutely devastating not to have an organization able to respond to the challenge.

We also learned how politicians can make things worse. States quarantining health workers when they returned from West Africa reduced the desire of experts to volunteer for service. When the US Department of Health and Human Services asked me for recommendations, I was able to include one facetious recommendation. Because the Republican governor of New Jersey and the Democratic governor of New York had both imposed unscientific rules on the quarantine of returnees who were not sick and only needed to have their temperatures checked each day, I suggested the federal government halt all flights out of those two states in an attempt to reduce the spread of political stupidity.

But there are also hopes. Perhaps we will now get the strong WHO the world needs—one without a board of 194 ministers of health and regional offices constantly trying to undercut headquarters in Geneva, a WHO that has an adequate budget, a way to reduce the political barriers to employment of the best people possible, and a mandate to follow the science rather than the politics.

Perhaps we will get a global United Nations synthesis that reduces the tension and antagonism between UN agencies intent on protecting their turf. This global health problem may have been required to force us all to look at the lessons of the past seventy years and ask if we can't do better.

chapter 4

A SHORT HISTORY OF THE CDC

The United States needed a CDC from the beginning but didn't know it. The country muddled through smallpox, cholera, malaria, and yellow fever without the national coordination that could have improved its response.

There are three essentials for good public health programs. The first is the conviction that the basis for public health is to achieve health equity; therefore, the bottom line is social justice in health. Second is the understanding that the science base is epidemiology. It is epidemiology that determines the gaps in social justice, identifies the groups with poor health outcomes, discovers the details of disease causation, and provides clues to how corrective action might improve health. The third essential is the need for good management for efficient implementation of corrective actions. I will assume that the first is a given. This chapter describes the development of epidemiology and management at the CDC.

Until 1950, not a single national surveillance program existed for any disease. While the principles of epidemiology were practiced wherever public health programs were implemented, no national leadership in epidemiology existed that states and counties could easily call on in times of need. That all changed in a relatively short period of time.

Epidemiology

John Snow is often called the Father of Epidemiology because of his study, published in 1849, in which he concluded that cholera was being spread by one of the providers of water in London and then pinpointed the Broad Street pump as a source of the problem. This was before the germ theory of disease was understood, so Snow's conclusion was based on what we now regard as epidemiologic evidence. It must have seemed flimsy to many, but when Snow removed the handle from the pump, the outbreak abated.

It was an important moment in the history of epidemiology. However, even before this episode Ignaz Semmelweiss, working at the Vienna General Hospital, was puzzled that the First Clinic, managed by doctors and his responsibility, had a higher rate of maternal mortality than the Second Clinic, managed by midwives. Puerperal fever following childbirth was usually the cause of death. Also known as "child bed fever," this infection is usually caused by *Staphylococcus* or *Streptococcus* organisms entering the uterus and then becoming systemic infections. Assigned to the obstetrical unit in July 1846, Semmelweiss began to ponder the different rates between the two clinics. He discovered that the differential risks were well known outside the hospital. The public understood that admissions were scheduled for twenty-four hours on one unit followed by twenty-four hours on the other unit. Women would attempt to either wait for admission, as long as possible during labor, or try for early admission in order to be admitted to the Second Clinic because of the lower risk of death (1).

The breakthrough in Semmelweiss's thinking came when a friend, Jakob Kolletschka, died after an accidental scalpel wound he incurred while conducting an autopsy. His symptoms resembled puerperal fever, the illness affecting women after childbirth. Semmelweiss concluded that doctors, who often conducted autopsies first thing in the morning, were transmitting something from the autopsy to the delivery room. Submicroscopic germs were not yet understood, but Semmelweiss was correct, and he instituted a handwashing policy, using a solution that contained calcium hypochlorite, between autopsy sessions and delivering babies. Mortality rates dropped from 18.3 percent in the First Clinic in April 1847 to 2.2 percent in June. This phenomenal breakthrough in observation was followed by the determination and interpretation of rates, the introduction of an intervention, and the subsequent saving of lives. So perhaps it would be appropriate to designate Semmelweiss as the Father of Epidemiology.

However, advances in epidemiology occurred even earlier than Semmelweiss's contributions. Oliver Wendell Holmes Sr., born in 1809, the same year as Abraham Lincoln, switched from law to medicine and spent formative years in Paris under the mentorship of Dr. Pierre Charles Alexandre Louis. Dr. Louis was an early clinical epidemiologist (which means he learned the subject from someone, despite the frequent assertion that Snow was the Father of Epidemiology), who demonstrated that bloodletting did not work. How many people were killed by draining blood is unknown, but finally Louis subjected the idea to study and found it wanting. He had a profound influence on Holmes, and Holmes published a paper in 1843 titled "The Contagiousness of Puerperal Fever" (2). Holmes postulated that physicians' unclean hands spread puerperal fever to patients. Hence, we have a new contender for the title of Father of Epidemiology—Holmes.

A half-century before Holmes's paper, Dr. Alexander Gordon published the *Treatise on the Epidemic of Puerperal Fever* (1795) (3). In his publication, he warns that the condition was transmitted from one case to another by midwives and doctors. He wrote, "It is a disagreeable declaration for me to mention, that I myself was the means of carrying the infection to a great number of women."

As Gordon was observing and writing his paper on puerperal fever, Edward Jenner was studying what happened to milkmaids during smallpox outbreaks. Jenner's mentor, John Hunter, had suggested the topic, and a milkmaid, now lost to history, had said to Jenner that she was protected from smallpox because she had experienced cowpox on her hands from milking cows. Jenner studied the experience of milkmaids who had acquired cowpox lesions in this manner and documented their protection from smallpox during subsequent smallpox outbreaks. As mentioned earlier, in 1796, he demonstrated the ability to provide this protection intentionally (4) by transmitting material from the cowpox lesion of a milkmaid, Sarah Nelmes, to a boy, James Phipps. Phipps developed a sore at the site of injection, and weeks later he was protected from a deliberate attempt to infect him with the smallpox virus.

The lesson may be that there is no true Father or Mother of Epidemiology. Rather, making observations to predict the future is as old as hunters, who improved their hunting success by observing and developing the equivalent of rates to compare the likelihood of success in different geographic areas and using various methods of hunting. Likewise, gatherers remembered the chances of finding roots or berries based on terrain, weather, and time of year. Rates were the unrecognized bottom line for those observations.

The people mentioned were all important in the history of epidemiology. But many other events, some known, most unknown, have improved the field of epidemiology.

One event was the establishment of the first school of public health in the United States in 1916 at Johns Hopkins University. Funded by a grant from the Rockefeller Foundation, it included the secondment of Wade Hampton Frost by the US Public Health Service to start a Department of Epidemiology. His experience with yellow fever, influenza, and tuberculosis provided real-world experiences in applied epidemiology. Frost later became the dean of the school.

The legacy of applied epidemiology was passed on to Alexander Langmuir, who received his training at Johns Hopkins before moving to the CDC in 1949. At the CDC, he encountered a workforce shaped by the war effort, the need to advise on tropical diseases in returning troops, and a new fear, the threat of an enemy using microorganisms for biological warfare. This was to lead to his greatest contribution: the corps of medical detectives known as the Epidemic Intelligence Service (EIS).

Malaria

When Langmuir arrived in 1949, the CDC was only three years old, having evolved from the Malaria Control Program, which started in 1942. The United States, in 1942, was rapidly gearing up to confront the demands of two simultaneous wars, one in Europe to meet the aggression of Germany, the other in the Pacific to counter the Japanese attack on Pearl Harbor. Military training camps were found throughout the country, but especially in the South, where temperate weather permitted more days of outdoor training.

The price for better weather was malaria. Malaria reduced recruit training time. Trainees from other parts of the United States had never been exposed to the disease. The United States responded with a malaria control program, headquartered in Atlanta, Georgia. One clear objective was the establishment of a one-mile malaria-free zone around every military base. Thousands of workers drained swamps, used insecticides, and learned about tropical diseases. And time lost to illness among the recruits was reduced.

Joe Mountin

The Malaria Control Program became a brain trust for malaria research and other tropical diseases plaguing troops in the Pacific and after their return home. At the beginning of the war, Dr. Joseph Mountin pushed to protect the 600 or so military bases from malaria. Mountin became a legend in public health, working in the US Public Health Service during World War I and continuing until his early death at age 61 in 1952. He became a passionate promoter of everything from chronic disease control to infectious disease programs and even to polar health. At the end of World War II, Mountin foresaw the need for a strong national center for communicable diseases. He successfully kept this unusual group of scientists together with a mandate that expanded to include the study and control of communicable diseases in general. The program became the Communicable Disease Center (CDC) on July 1, 1946.

Mountin was a man of unusual vision. He not only saw the future of the CDC but also recognized the importance of epidemiology—hence, the arrival of Langmuir. Mountin also foresaw the role of chronic diseases in public health and initiated the Framingham Study in 1948. Much of what we know about heart disease and the role of diet, exercise, and medications comes from this continuing, long-term longitudinal study of a single community. Mountin may not have anticipated it, but the CDC eventually expanded its scope from infectious diseases to the broad spectrum of public health, including chronic diseases.

Langmuir's arrival increased the emphasis on epidemiology, which he once described as simply acquiring a numerator and a denominator, developing a rate, and acquiring enough information to accurately understand that rate. While he was a driving force in epidemiology in general, his lasting legacy was the program mentioned earlier, the EIS. An outbreak of hemorrhagic fever in troops during the Korean War underscored the immediate need for persons trained in detecting, understanding, and responding to epidemics. The United States was concerned that China had intentionally released Korean hemorrhagic fever, but we later learned that China had increased its virology programs, fearing the United States had released the virus.

In any case, a tradition was born. The dedication of the Alexander Langmuir Auditorium at the CDC in 2011 provided an opportunity both to honor Langmuir and to recall his approach. He was simultaneously respected, adored, and feared. Articles by EIS officers, intended for publication in the medical literature, were sent back to subordinates by Langmuir time after time for revisions in order "to get it right." The demands were balanced by his personal interest in the EIS officers. After presenting at the annual EIS conference (where current officers presented interesting outbreak investigations and were then subjected to a question-and-answer session), most officers shared the anxiety of having Langmuir stand to ask a question that went to the heart of the issue and had often been overlooked by the presenter.

The approach worked, and the eagerness to please Langmuir caused the EIS officers to become professional in a very short time. At the dedication of the auditorium, one of his granddaughters was a final speaker. She related that after his retirement, Langmuir would arrange a family dinner in Atlanta every year, at the time of the EIS conference. To her he was a grandfather, and she could not even fathom that grown people at the CDC would quake in his presence.

A strong EIS became part of the genetic code that formed the CDC of today. Because it was a way to fulfill a draft obligation for young men, many more applied than could be accepted, and Langmuir could be selective in his choices. Many of those selected found the work intriguing and made a vocation of public health even though they had planned to return after their two-year stint to other careers.

The assignment of EIS officers to states, cities, and universities provided the CDC with a direct connection to the field concerns of public health. Many of those assigned continued training in public health and worked with the CDC in state, county, and university positions. A trust developed between states and the CDC that may be unique in the annals of the federal government.

Langmuir's vision of an EIS also had an effect on the CDC itself. To support this cadre of field epidemiologists, the CDC had to upgrade its abilities and have staff of the highest caliber. It needed to truly be the gold standard for public health practice and public health laboratory capabilities. It was forced into greatness.

Over time this truth was recognized, and epidemiology was used to define and measure health problems and to suggest responses. So epidemiology became important largely because of the driving force of Langmuir.

How did management become a priority? Largely by chance. Without great forethought or planning, the CDC was blessed by the unexpected development of a managerial cadre as the result of people who were concentrating on a specific cluster of diseases rather than the CDC in general.

Public Health Advisors

Following World War II, Johannes Stuart, an economist working in the Venereal Disease Division of the Public Health Service, was charged with developing a program to treat and reduce the spread of sexually transmitted diseases, especially syphilis. He organized a program that employed carefully selected college graduates, who were taught to trace the contacts of people with sexually transmitted diseases and enroll them in treatment programs. A skeptical supervisor allowed him to institute a pilot program with six young college graduates in 1948. Great diplomatic and psychological skills were required to induce people to provide information on their sexual partners. And detective skills were required to find those sexual contacts, especially if they involved one-night stands. Unusual tenacity was also required. The program was successful, and its Washington, DC, headquarters was moved to the CDC after the CDC became recognized for its work in public health.

The most successful syphilis detectives were those with the best management and people skills, and they soon attracted the attention of those in charge of other public health programs at the CDC. Over time, venereal disease workers (officially known as public health advisors) were managing vaccine, tuberculosis, and smallpox programs. Indeed, it was the experience of surveillance and containment in the field of sexually transmitted diseases that proved so useful in smallpox eradication.

William "Bill" Watson, one of the first members of the group, eventually became the deputy director of the CDC. Bill had left for war as a young and capable product of rural South Carolina. His experiences included capture by the Germans and time in a prisoner of war camp outside of Dresden. He saw the bombing of that city and the destruction made famous by Kurt Vonnegut in his book *Slaughterhouse-Five*. Bill wrote his own book of his experiences, entitled *First Class Privates*. Bill Watson was revered as a leader and manager, and when the professional managers at the CDC (i.e., the public health advisors) organized to improve mutual support, they called themselves the Watsonian Society.

Location (Location, Location)

The importance of epidemiology and management is straightforward. But why is the CDC located next to Emory University?

There is a history to everything. The CEO of Coca-Cola, Robert Woodruff, had made a commitment to have Coca-Cola available wherever US troops were stationed during World War II. This stance later provided the company with overseas bottling plants that immensely benefited global expansion. It also resulted in a friendship between Woodruff and General Dwight D. Eisenhower. In the postwar years, Woodruff became a member of President Eisenhower's golf clique, made up of some of the most powerful men in the nation. The press referred to this group as "Ike's Millionaires."

Woodruff also had close connections with Emory and served on the Emory board of trustees from 1935 to 1948. Starting in 1937, Woodruff began giving money to Emory for a series of buildings (seven by 2014) and programs, and he later provided Emory with a gift of $105 million to expand and deepen its capacity in higher education.

A plantation owned by Woodruff had a continuous problem with malaria. Mountin soon became part of the Woodruff network, advising him on the latest knowledge about malaria control.

With the establishment of the CDC, Woodruff saw an opportunity to merge some of his interests. A fifteen-acre plot of land on Clifton Road, next to Emory, seemed to him the ideal place for the CDC. In 1947, Woodruff arranged to have it sold for $1 to the government and waited for his dream to be fulfilled. He was not acquainted with the long process of government planning, appropriations, and everything else involved, and he became impatient. Woodruff finally called President Eisenhower and got him on a golf course in Denver. (This, before any of us had cell phones.) He asked the president if he had paper and pencil and got an affirmative. He then said that he had given land to Emory to give to the government to build the headquarters for the CDC, but nothing was happening. Eisenhower told him he would be happy to check into it and asked for a paragraph on the details to be sent to him. Woodruff supposedly responded, "That is why I asked if you had paper and pencil." Soon bulldozers were on the property and building began (5).

The CDC headquarters on Clifton Road became institutionalized as the only Public Health Service agency with headquarters outside of the Washington, DC, area. Its later prominence around the world as the standard for public health owes much to a succession of incredibly gifted and superb scientists, but it was undoubtedly aided by Woodruff, who was able to ensure that the CDC was a safe distance from the fumbling hands of Washington, DC's politicians.

Science Revolution

A scientific revolution occurred in the twentieth century, mostly in our understanding of physics. There are still mysteries to be sure, but, in general, a century after Albert Einstein's paper on relativity, the God Particle had been demonstrated and the basic laws of physics had been established. There are no shortages of areas to be explored in understanding the universe, parallel universes, and the like, but the foundations of physics on this planet have generally been set.

In biology, however, understanding lagged by fifty to one hundred years. However, the twenty-first century will be known as the century of biology. When Francis H. Crick died at age 88, I found myself contemplating the speed of biological progress in his lifetime. It was in April 1953 that he and James Watson reported on their understanding of the double helix. I was just graduating from high school, where I was taught there were twenty-four pairs of chromosomes for humans rather than twenty-three. Crick and Watson now provided new insights into the genetic transmission of life. In the past fifty years, we have therefore gone from not even knowing how many chromosomes there are in a human to a catalog of the millions of amino acids in the first complete human genome. We have not only learned about the four-letter alphabet that contains the secrets of all species known in the history of the world, but we have also begun to write compositions using that alphabet. This permits the possibility of altering insect vectors so they cannot transmit human diseases, altering microorganisms in the development of vaccines, and providing rapid and accurate diagnostic techniques. It may even permit treatment of chronic conditions or cancers by attaching DNA segments to microorganisms that seek out the cancer or specific deficits, such as those found in muscular dystrophy. The possibilities are as challenging to understand as the universe itself.

I had the chance to meet and talk with Francis Crick at the Salk Institute in 2002, a year after I met James Watson. For a public health practitioner, these were significant events. Crick was in that elite group of geniuses who see through to solutions even outside their fields. He continued to contribute until his death. It is said that he was always gracious and humble; yet James Watson starts his book *The Double Helix* by saying, "I have never seen Francis Crick in a modest mood" (6). Whatever the truth, CDC owes much to these two men.

The Role of Emory University

The world and the CDC would benefit in this developing scientific explosion by its close association with an academic community. However, Woodruff's dream of a real connection between the CDC and Emory took decades to develop. While the relationship was cordial, it did not reach a lift-off stage. The development of an Emory program in community health, which matured into a school of public health, provided the vehicle. But critical mass was finally achieved when a dean of the school was recruited from the CDC. Dean Jim Curran had headed up the HIV-AIDS program at the CDC. He provided an extraordinary calming effect on this volatile problem and strolled with confidence and deliberation through the minefields. Clinical medicine, public health, and medical research all saw themselves as the owners of the problem. Jim could converse with all of them. The gay and straight communities were often pitted against each other, but he was accepted by both. Friction between gay communities and communities of color provided some of the toughest problems in the late 1980s, but in his willingness to engage all, Dr. Curran was seen as a leader.

The search committee that recommended Dr. Curran for the position recognized his qualities, but not all were comfortable with a CDC person at Emory. A few resented the fact that the CDC would often get national or international publicity. But when the decision was made, no one ever looked back with regret. The Emory School of Public Health, at a very young age, became one of the leaders in public health education and then in global health education. During the Ebola outbreak in West Africa in 2015, the value of this relationship was highlighted. Twelve years earlier, the CDC had provided Emory with funds to develop a treatment center capable of treating diseases such as Ebola. When the time came for treating volunteers who had become infected in Africa, Emory was prepared to provide superb care. In addition, the Emory Eye Center deployed experts to West Africa to care for Ebola survivors with eye complications of Ebola.

Woodruff would be very pleased.

chapter 5

THE FEARS OF THE RICH
AND THE NEEDS OF THE POOR

Life plans are an illusion. I tell students that they cannot imagine the opportunities that life will present and that they should spend their time developing a life philosophy rather than a life plan.

My life plan was to work in Africa. I had no idea that a two-year stint at the CDC, fulfilling a draft obligation, would capture me for life. I did not know that the EIS program would be one of the best mechanisms yet devised to propel people into global health. I entered this portal through good fortune, not through careful analysis, and only in retrospect realize the role of a mentor in providing this experience—an experience that provides one perspective on the CDC.

I also did not know that epidemiology would be the science base for everything done in public health or that we all use epidemiology daily but unconsciously. We develop our own risk comparisons, both to avoid unpleasant situations or to enhance pleasant ones. Dopamine levels influence how much risk we seek or avoid. We try to avoid contacts with bullies, who might beat us up, and so we observe their habits and know where they are likely to be. We arrange, but make it appear to be by chance, to run into a girl we are hoping to meet. It isn't chance because we have observed the route she takes walking home from school or when she goes to the library. Epidemiology is a daily companion, even if we're not aware of it.

Looking back, I now see that I deliberately used the skills of an epidemiologist to get a driver's license. I passed my sixteenth birthday in a body cast, the result of a hip injury, and expected to get my driver's license immediately on release from the cast. I was mistaken. My left knee was frozen in extension, and my left ankle had limited mobility. I was told I would never walk again without crutches.

That only fueled my desire for freedom, and soon I was walking without crutches and could focus on getting a driver's license. The problem with the limited movement in my left leg joints meant that I had to operate the clutch, brake pedal, and accelerator with my right foot. It can be done but with a certain amount of jerkiness in getting started. An automatic transmission would have made it easy, but that is not what we had. The clutch must be released slowly to avoid a stall; the right foot then shifts from the clutch to the accelerator. I could easily go from first to second to third gears without using the clutch, by moving the shifter to neutral and increasing the motor speed so the transmission would mesh. It was only the initial start that was awkward. I could drive safely and would automatically shift into neutral as I put on the brakes, but there was no way I could have passed a road test with an examiner in the car.

Driver's licenses were awarded once a week in Colville, Washington. A state patrolman would come to our town and give the written and driving tests. I knew the driving manual by heart, but I went to the weekly session on the pretext of getting a book to study. I sat down and pretended to read the book while I watched to see if there were any possible ways to avoid the actual driving part of the test.

Applicants would be given a written test at the counter. They then sat at one of the half-dozen tables to take the test. It was returned to the examiner, and, after grading, the patrolman would take the applicants for the driving test. The license would be issued, and the next applicant would be seen. I noticed, during the middle of the afternoon, when a half-dozen people completed their tests at about the same time, that the patrolman skipped the driving test.

Years later I realized I was practicing epidemiology. The rate (or risk) of a driving test was 100 percent if only one person was in line to have his or her test graded. But the rate (or risk) of a driving test declined when there were others waiting to have their tests graded and declined precipitously when the line was long. So the plan was to get in a long line but be near the head of that line.

The next week I stayed outside the room until a group of people came for their licenses. I entered in their midst, completed the test quickly, and then watched until I saw that four or five were almost finished with the test. I went to the examiner's desk near the front of the group, with a line forming behind me. Sure enough, within minutes I had a license without taking the driving test. Epidemiology works!

The Lure of the CDC

When J. D. (Don) Millar called me in early 1962 to say that I had been accepted into the EIS program, it changed my career trajectory. I had already been accepted into an internal medicine residency program, but by this time, I was reading the various publications from the WHO and becoming increasingly interested in global health. (Although then it was always referred to as international health or tropical medicine.) There were various ways to get into global health in those days, but few were straightforward. There was little job security and to say there was not much competition is an understatement. Few faculty members at my medical school, other than Rei Ravenholt, had an interest in the subject. At my fiftieth medical school class reunion, a classmate confessed that when I told him I wanted to go into global health, he said to himself, *What a waste.*

The lack of competition was matched by a paucity of good financial pathways. In those days, every person going into global health cut his or her own path through the morass. It later became clear that one of the few truly good pathways was through joining the EIS. Not only did that program make it possible to become acquainted with people and programs with global interests but also the experiences that made the CDC a gold standard for public health in the United States soon made it a gold standard for global health. Once again, without a clear personal plan, and with little understanding that the EIS was a great career development move for global health, the decision to join the EIS turned out to be career changing.

EIS was developed by Dr. Alex Langmuir in 1951, as mentioned earlier, as a response to concerns that Korean hemorrhagic fever might have been introduced deliberately during the Korean conflict. It had not been, but the fear alone led to one of the most important developments in public health history. This fact reinforced a bias that I developed over the years when resources were so scarce in global health, namely, that the way to improve health equity is to figure out how to *link the fears of the rich to the needs of the poor.* The rich will respond to AIDS, to Ebola, to drug-resistant tuberculosis, to bioterrorism, because they realize they stand to benefit, as they also are at risk. But it is much more difficult to get them to respond to river blindness, intestinal worms, or even malaria because they don't feel the threat to themselves. Vaccines in the United States are purchased for all because the powerful realize we are all at risk. For many years, I had told students that Ebola could be one such link, and 2014 proved that point.

To train a group of people to respond to bioterrorism required training them in the common health outbreaks that involve the United States every day. Originally, that meant infectious diseases. Because bioterrorism involved the very security of the country, EIS officers were recruited as military officers, and the two-year program satisfied military draft requirements. One implication of this is that originally all EIS officers were men, as women were not subject to the draft. Another implication was that officers were expected to wear uniforms, thereby making it clear that two personnel systems were involved at the CDC, the Civil Service and the Commissioned Corps. This dress code was accepted at the Pentagon and other places with military and civilian employees, but it often confused people in public health. (It also inspired longtime health educator Hod Ogden to write lyrics for a song, indicating that bureaucrats in Washington, DC, when dealing with the CDC, were "Civil to the servants, but rotten to the Corps.") Another implication of the draft recruitment was that, while most originally entered to satisfy military service, many found the work so interesting that they became public health workers for life.

A matching process was used in assigning new EIS officers. They were expected to attend the EIS conference, held each April at the CDC, preceding the initiation of their employment in July. They attended the conference meetings but also interviewed with programs with openings for EIS officers. At the end of the week, prospective officers listed the programs they would prefer in priority order. The programs also listed the EIS officers they would like assigned to them in priority order. Most officers and programs got one of their top-three selections.

As a medical student, I had worked for Rei Ravenholt, an early EIS officer, and at the time the epidemiologist for Seattle-King County. He had a high energy level, an infectious interest in a wide variety of subjects, and boldness in taking on anyone, whether the tobacco companies' causing enormous harm or his fellow physicians' causing hospital infections. He was always embroiled in controversy but appeared to relish the battle. He was generous with his time to talk about public health issues requiring attention, exuded charisma, and attracted a group of students to help him in his many research projects. He was an enthusiastic promoter of the EIS, and I am grateful that his descriptions caught my interest.

The Value of Available Resources

As a medical student, two projects especially interested me. One was a review of death certificates in Seattle, to understand changing patterns of death classifications and disease in the history of the city. For example, it was possible to get some idea of the role of fatalities due to *Staphylococcus* organisms by knowing the various names given to staph infections over the years. Or it was possible to plot the change in causes of death due to violence; for example, deaths due to elevator accidents went down as elevators became safer, while automobile deaths went up.

But it was also possible to plot the increased role of tobacco as a cause of early death. The increase in lung cancer deaths led to my first paper in a peer-reviewed journal, as we looked at the life expectancy of patients following a diagnosis of lung cancer (1). The discouraging summary was that there had been little progress in treating lung cancer in thirty years, and the increases in life span after diagnosis were generally the result of earlier diagnosis rather than clinical success in treatment. Few patients survived five years after diagnosis, a disheartening situation. With a diagnosis of lung cancer, no matter how much money a person had, he or she would have traded it all to go back three decades to change smoking habits.

Individuals, cities, states, nations, and the world have a predictable quality: they do not value health until they lose it. The job of public health is to try and rewrite history *before* it happens. And that is not easy. Prevention is such a sensible approach that one thinks it should be in great demand. I had no idea how hard it would be in practice.

EIS Training

The EIS program developed some approaches that remain even sixty years later. Many officers were assigned to states, as that is where epidemic investigations often begin. Some were assigned to universities or other federal agencies, and many were assigned to the CDC headquarters in Atlanta or one of its branch offices. Regardless of assignment, all EIS officers returned to Atlanta for a week in April to present interesting cases and to participate in the interrogation of other officers presenting cases at the EIS conference. Rigid rules prevailed—such as no presentation longer than ten minutes, followed by ten-minute question periods—and have stood the test of time. But on Thursday nights, the rules relaxed. The outgoing class would perform a skit. It was a chance to ridicule the program, supervisors, and approaches, playing the role of jesters to the EIS. I always contended that this is when the EIS creativity was most in evidence.

An additional tradition developed. EIS officers remained in the club forever. An annual compilation was published summarizing the career of each officer, where he or she had lived, language abilities, professional expertise, and family information. With this *EIS Directory*, it was possible to quickly call on past officers for special problems that used their skills. Interestingly, many former officers returned for the EIS conference at their own expense, simply because the experience was so rich, and it provided an annual summary of public health problems.

Eventually, the target of investigations went beyond infectious diseases to include chronic diseases, injuries, natural disasters, nutrition, occupational and environmental problems, famine, and even homicides. When the military draft was formally lifted, the program began to recruit women, and now most classes are more than 50 percent female. While the original officers were predominantly physicians, veterinarians, and statisticians, diversity soon developed to include anthropologists, sociologists, and, indeed, most professions.

My first EIS conference in 1962 was a changing point in my life. Becoming an EIS officer was more than simply a new position. I liked the people. They were social activists, committed to solving the health problems of whole populations. The conference was stimulating, the presentations dealt with current problems, and the discussions were animated. After multiple interviews, I made my first choice, a state assignment to Colorado. It provided exposure to a spectrum of public health problems. The downside, of course, was not becoming a cutting-edge expert in a specific area, such as respiratory infections, diarrheal disease, or unusual pathogens.

June 30 was my last day as an intern, and my wife, Paula, and I drove from New York to Atlanta. Paula was quite pregnant, and our excitement was boundless.

July 1962 was my training period before going to Colorado. Paula and I got an efficiency apartment within a block of the famed Fox Theater in Atlanta, and I took the bus each day to the CDC. The lectures were compelling, and the afternoons were taken up with problems, such as discussing and solving previous outbreaks from the public health records, with information provided in the sequence it was first known to the original investigators. Statistical problems were presented, and I participated in a field exercise to collect information from a sample of houses visited in Atlanta, followed by analysis of the information obtained. It was all very practical.

As a fourth-year medical student at the University of Washington, I had attended a class in public health practice taught by Russ Alexander. He had been an EIS officer, and he used one of the outbreak presentations that he encountered at the CDC for my medical school class. It was an outbreak of pellagra, but that fact was not known to the students in the beginning. The seasonality, age distribution, rates by socioeconomic status, death rates, and the like all appeared to be caused by an infectious disease. So it was a surprise, during the discussion, to find that the cause of the outbreak was a nutritional deficiency. I was equally surprised, during the EIS course, to have the same problem presented. The difference was that I could ask great questions because I now knew the rest of the story. Some forty years later, I introduced Russ for a talk he was giving, and I could now thank him. By looking good during this exercise at the EIS course, I was incorrectly labeled as having keen insight rather than having average memory.

Throughout the course, the academic presentations were interspersed with real-time reports on ongoing investigations. Sometimes this was a call from the officer in the field or a summary of the outbreak investigation by the supervisor in Atlanta. When the training program was completed, Langmuir called us together to brief us on the latest news. He filled us in on the Sabin oral polio vaccine, a major advancement in the attempt to control polio. Given by mouth, it avoided the trauma of an injection and could be given by anyone. However, early evaluation was showing that it could also cause polio in some recipients or in the contacts of recipients. The CDC was still trying to estimate the level of risk but felt it might be a case of polio for every 1 million to 2 million children receiving the vaccine. Therefore, parents and providers should have this information as they made decisions on the use of the vaccine, Langmuir said. I had no idea at the time that this would be a contentious issue in Colorado and even more so in later years with the global effort to eradicate polio.

Assignment to Denver

When Paula and I departed for Denver in August, she was close to her delivery date. It is the hubris of youth and inexperience that made our traveling at this time possible. I had delivered twenty-eight babies during my month on OB/GYN, some months earlier, and so felt comfortable with the idea of delivering another one.

When we arrived in Denver, our first stop was Fitzsimmons Army Hospital to make an appointment at the obstetrics clinic. Only after that task was completed, did we check into a motel. We were still staying in the motel when Paula's contractions started early one morning. On the way to the hospital, we stopped at a drugstore. I picked up a paperback titled *Man-eaters of Kumaon* by Jim Corbett. (Eleven years later we would go to the Corbett Park in India and from the back of an elephant attempt to see a tiger in the area where Corbett had been a game warden.)

The contractions continued and despite a scare with toxemia of pregnancy, David was born that evening. By 5 the next morning, Paula was up making her own bed. (Military hospitals have strict rules.) David's first home after the hospital was a motel room, and his bed was a dresser drawer.

The EIS position in Colorado was close to ideal. My supervisor, Cecil Mollahan, was a bright and conscientious epidemiologist. He had an MPH from the Harvard School of Public Health and had grown up in Colorado, so he had an understanding of the state. Although Cecil could not always contain his affinity for alcohol, he was conscientious and would often start the day with a review of some of the problems I might encounter in the late afternoon if I alone would have to make the decisions. This unusual approach to supervising not only gave me greater responsibility and input from a savvy person but also gave me an insight into addiction in the best of people.

Within weeks I had investigated malaria in a person returning from Africa and a small outbreak of typhoid fever in Center, Colorado, which we traced to a grandmother who was a typhoid carrier. Center is located in South Park. To enter South Park from the north and suddenly see the vista of a flat valley at 10,000 feet, surrounded by peaks going up to 14,000 feet, was absolutely breathtaking. Who could have believed such beauty? This joy came despite being accustomed to seeing Mt. Rainier, the Cascades, and the Olympics during college and graduate school. I bought a book on ghost towns of Colorado, and on my many trips, I would make side visits to one or more of these remnants of mining days.

The medical society asked me to address them on the problems of polio vaccine. When I explained the risks of disease associated with the oral polio vaccine, I was surprised by the strong and repeated assertion that the risk was low and need not be conveyed to parents. I was being challenged on my assertion that although the risk was low, it was nevertheless real, and therefore had to be shared with recipients, even if that made immunization programs more difficult. To my surprise and relief, Gordon Meiklejohn stood up to defend my argument. Gordon was well respected and the head of the Internal Medicine Department at the University of Colorado Medical School. With his endorsement, medical society members changed their views and supported transparency with parents. Throughout my time in

Colorado, Gordon was an interested participant in infectious disease problems. In later years, he became heavily involved in smallpox eradication and spent time in India as a short-term special epidemiologist.

The years in Colorado were good years. The work was interesting, and my appreciation of the CDC continued to grow as the people there were always available for advice and help in investigations.

Encountering Smallpox

I developed an interest in smallpox while investigating a suspected smallpox case in Farmington, New Mexico. Less than a year after entering the EIS, the April 1963 EIS conference led to an unusual opportunity. An announcement was made at the conference that the Peace Corps physician in India had to leave because of illness, and the Peace Corps was looking for a three-month volunteer to fill the position while they recruited for a new physician. I applied and spent a busy few weeks of orientation before departing for India.

Preparations included getting vaccination boosters and personal medications for malaria prophylaxis and common respiratory and gastrointestinal illnesses. I reviewed the most common medical problems encountered by Peace Corps volunteers. I traveled to Washington, DC, for interviews and briefings on India and the Peace Corps, bought books on the history of India, and reviewed papers on the disease patterns and medical care systems in the country. In recent years, the Internet has made it possible to collect any information you need after you enter a country. However, in the early 1960s, you had to predict what information you would want and take it with you. For the three months of my assignment, I was always scrambling to get information on diseases or treatments that I had overlooked in my preparations. And there is no way to prepare for the heat in India in May.

The Peace Corps was still new and finding its way. The Peace Corps country representative for India was Charles Houston. I had gone to India to do a job, not to acquire yet another unusual mentor. But acquire one I did. Although a cardiologist by background, Houston had vast interests, among them climbing K2, the second highest mountain on Earth (2). He was a hero to the climbing community because of his attempt, in 1953, to rescue a K2 climber with deep vein thrombosis during a storm. An exceptional team of climbers had been within striking distance of the summit but turned back without an argument to aid a sick person. The climber did not survive, but the very audacity of trying to execute this mission in a storm left climbers astounded. It was this leadership quality—including Houston's ability to diagnose a problem, develop a response, get others to follow, and then show such tenacity that no one could shirk his or her responsibility—that made him such a successful leader in climbing, in medicine, and in inspiring Peace Corps volunteers in India.

In India, I could test my interest in tropical diseases and international health. At Houston's urging, I visited hospitals, made rounds, treated volunteers, and arranged for sick Peace Corps volunteers to be hospitalized for major illnesses. I was invited into the homes of local staff and introduced to foods, culture, beliefs, and variety that make India one of the most compelling places in the world to work. Traveling by train to an unfamiliar area in order to locate a Peace Corps volunteer was an adventure in navigation. Before smartphones and GPS devices, one had to find someone who knew about an American in the area. Without fail, there was always someone who could direct me to someone who might know. Without advertising it, the CDC was showing itself to be a global agency, providing a pathway for those interested in global health.

While much of my time was spent on Peace Corps health matters, there were adventures. While visiting volunteers working on poultry projects in the Terai area of Uttar Pradesh, I learned of a new agricultural expansion that was taking place. While the term *Terai* originally referred to wetlands, it now described the plains bordering the Siwalik Hills. Parts of the Terai included recently deforested areas and thus were close to the wildlife of the forest.

Leaving the guesthouse where I had stayed overnight, I was told the volunteers were at the farm of a wealthy Punjabi farmer. The farmer's yard contained about two dozen people, all talking about the man-eating tiger that had been spotted that morning. Corbett's book *Man-eaters of Kumaon* had introduced me to both this area of India and the problem of tigers' preying on people. Generally, only tigers with physical disabilities that make it difficult to hunt their regular game will prey on humans. Corbett is still remembered in India for killing dozens of proven man-eaters, often after they had killed dozens and in some cases even hundreds of people. A tiger had often eluded other hunters by the time Corbett was called in, and he would hunt alone, on foot, relentlessly tracking and finally killing the tiger.

The tiger now in question had killed several farmers in the area and was much feared. The group gathered that morning was drinking beer and developing a plan. (The beer, evidently, made the plan seem increasingly possible.) The Punjabi farmer had a number of large, Russian-built tractors and decided to have men with guns sit on the large fenders and stand on the various bars at the back of the tractors. The men would then traverse the fields, hoping to flush out the tiger, allowing one of the men a shot. I was invited to climb on one of the tractors to observe. I was too stupid and too curious to refuse.

With everyone loaded on the tractors, the signal was given to begin. The tractor drivers, accustomed to pulling loads, accelerated with the usual power, but with no load the front wheels left the ground, and everyone fell off the back of the tractors into a heap of bodies with guns sticking out of the pile. None of the guns fired, and everyone reassembled, and the tractors accelerated more gently. Fortunately, the tiger was not sighted, reducing the chance that the hunters would inflict serious harm on one another. Only then could we get to the real reason for my visit, which was to assess their health status, administer gamma globulin as a protection against hepatitis, plan for their next trips to Delhi, and collect information on the results of their poultry and agriculture projects to provide to Charlie Houston.

Colorado Cases

After three exhilarating months in India, a new Peace Corps physician arrived, and I returned to my EIS position in Colorado.

As with most people my age, I recall exactly what I was doing when I learned that President John F. Kennedy had been assassinated. I was working on hepatitis statistics in my Denver office. I went home and, for the next few days, joined the rest of the country in watching television and wishing it were possible to reverse time.

My two-year assignment in Colorado flew by. One undertaking involved following children in Colorado Springs who had been vaccinated with a killed measles vaccine. Jonas Salk had demonstrated that recipients of a killed polio vaccine developed antibodies. Then, Dr. Tommy Francis conducted a huge field trial on 1.8 million children with hundreds of thousands of volunteers to show, in less than two years, that the vaccine not only produced antibodies but also protected against the poliovirus. It was an exciting moment in medicine.

A few years later, there were similar hopes that a killed measles vaccine could protect against measles disease. A trial was conducted in Colorado Springs and indeed the vaccine elicited antibodies. Hopes were high, but then complications developed in some children if they were exposed to wild measles in later years. Some children were protected, but others developed what appeared to be an allergic response. While none of them died, it was clear that the vaccine could not be used on a mass basis. The results were published in an article I cowrote with Drs. Vince Fulginiti and C. Henry Kempe (3). The vaccine was dropped in favor of live measles vaccine.

Hepatitis outbreaks were constant in the 1960s, when there were no tests for the virus or antibodies. Cases were designated as A, B, or non-AB, based on clinical and epidemiologic findings. One memorable outbreak occurred in Minturn, Colorado, a small town near what would later be the Vail ski complex. An outbreak of hepatitis had frightened the community. There had been no deaths, but the lack of appetite, the yellow eyes, and the lack of energy led to concern. Some residents criticized the mayor, blaming him for a faulty water supply, which they felt had led to the outbreak. There was talk of impeachment.

In one of my more satisfying outbreak investigations, I collected information on the names of people with a history of hepatitis. As I was in a small town, I was able to interview many of them within a few hours. Hepatitis A, the most common type of hepatitis in Colorado, has an incubation period of two to four weeks but usually closer to four weeks. A common-source outbreak, such as a contaminated water supply, would have resulted in a cluster of onset dates about four weeks after the water supply became contaminated. However, if hepatitis A had spread from person to person, that would have supported disease-onset dates spread over an extended time period. It was quickly evident that the outbreak did not have a common source but was spreading through the community person to person. The grateful mayor's reputation was saved. This appreciation is about as close as public health people come to the expressions of gratitude that personal physicians routinely get.

The Jet Injector

In 1964, I was part of a CDC group that went to Tonga to test smallpox vaccine by using jet injectors. The armed forces had pioneered the use of jet injectors for needleless injections. They had then developed a small injector that required no electricity. Between injections, the injector was cocked by means of a foot-operated hydraulic pump.

The question to be studied in Tonga was, what dilution of vaccine could be used in jet injectors to obtain comparable take rates to those obtained with a multiple-pressure technique? The multiple-pressure approach involved a drop of vaccine on the skin and multiple depressions through the vaccine with a needle tangential to the skin surface. If performed correctly, the needle was intended to prick the skin on the upstroke, providing a small injury for the virus to begin multiplication. Success rates varied widely, and even the same person would have better success on some days than on others. The jet injector was a marked improvement in both speed and ability to replicate results between vaccinators and even at different times with the same vaccinator. It also had the advantage of reducing the vaccine usage since one-tenth of a milliliter (300 doses per ounce) was injected between the layers of the skin (intradermal), thus avoiding the usual wastage of vaccine.

A half-dozen CDC people, led by Dr. Ron Roberto, tried different dilutions and then read the results days after the vaccinations had been given by inspecting the injection site for the signs of virus multiplication that led to a distinct ulcer or pustule. Tonga was an ideal site because it had not used smallpox vaccine for many decades. (Thus, there was no interference in interpreting vaccination results.) The bottom line was that the method was reliable and allowed more than 100 million smallpox vaccinations to be conducted in West and Central Africa only a few years later.

It was an idyllic assignment. Tourism had not yet reached Tonga so there were no commercial hotels. The population lived up to the name given by Captain James Cook: the Friendly Islands. Villages would often prepare feasts to thank us for vaccinating. We would sit on the ground with a long table of banana leaves containing pork, vegetables, fruits of all kinds—and an elaborate ceremony. A young girl would be placed at the side of each visitor to keep our banana leaves piled high with food. Our previous work in schools, where we were provided cafeteria lunches, paled in comparison.

Queen Salote, a tall woman of regal bearing, was adored by her subjects. She had been queen since 1918 and continued until her death in 1965, a year after our smallpox studies. She invited us for a reception at the palace, where she showed us a tortoise given to the King of Tonga in 1777 by Captain Cook on his third voyage. It had been living in the Royal Palace ever since and was written up, with a picture, in *National Geographic*. It was another brush with history.

My two-year stint as an EIS officer was ending, and I was making plans for more training before leaving for Africa to run a medical program. Reflecting on those years, there are several lessons that shine through.

The EIS experience provides one of the best imaginable relationships between federal and state agencies. The assigned person answers to a

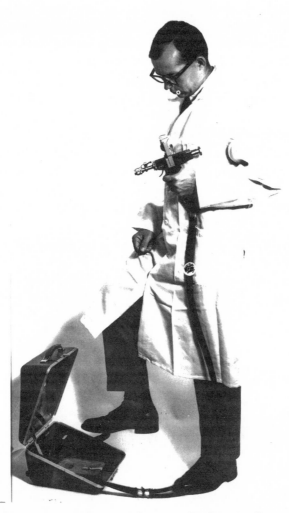

Ped-O-Jet demonstration by Dr. William H. "Bill" Stewart (Epidemic Intelligence Service class of 1951), 1966. Photo from the CDC

supervisor at the state but is available when needed for federal investigations. The state is provided with expertise and a direct channel to the CDC that it might not be able to have otherwise. The CDC, in turn, has a relationship that provides immediate access to health problems that it might not learn about so quickly were an EIS officer not on site.

State health officers offer another lesson. During my EIS assignment, Dr. Roy Cleere, the Colorado health officer, had been in the position for several decades and knew the state well. He became the interface between the scientific community and the political community. In later years, most state health officers were changed when a new governor was elected. The average length of stay in the position has now declined to three years or less. That the office is heavily based on politics rather than on public health has contributed to the weakening of the US public health system.

Then there is the lesson of informal networks. The short, two-year period in the EIS program provided an informal network, one that now encompasses more than 3,000 people. Throughout counties, states, academic institutions, foundations, federal agencies, and global institutions, finding a former EIS officer provides immediate rapport and common experiences. It is one of the strongest professional bonds I have experienced, exceeding that of medical school or other training programs. Fortunately, the approach is now being replicated in many countries.

chapter 6

BALANCING BABIES AND THE MARKETPLACE

Alex Langmuir often said that time imperatives sometimes required throwing EIS officers into the water. If they were unable to swim, they needed to know that there was a rescue team behind them.

The EIS training program always started as early as possible in July. By the end of the month, the fresh officers were dispatched to their new assignments.

One day short of the new assignments, on July 26, 1979, the Birth Defects Branch of the CDC received a report from a pediatric nephrologist in Memphis, Tennessee, of three cases of Bartter syndrome. This rare condition is caused by an autosomal recessive genetic condition that causes children to lose large amounts of sodium and potassium through their kidneys. This leads to a clinical syndrome known as metabolic alkalosis.

Only nine cases of Bartter syndrome had been reported in the world; therefore, the average pediatrician had never seen a child with the condition. Indeed, most pediatricians would never even hear the syndrome mentioned during training.

Normally, you simply cannot divert the short time available in a residency program to discuss issues that will never be seen. But surprisingly, Dr. Jose Cordero, an incoming EIS officer who would report for duty the next day, had actually treated one of those nine patients during his training at Boston City Hospital.

Cordero would have been an outstanding EIS officer even in the absence of this outbreak. Bright and hardworking, he threw himself into his work. However, this report immediately launched his EIS career. In Memphis, he found that all three children were less than 1 year old, had low potassium, low chloride, and metabolic alkalosis. Was this consistent with a diagnosis of Bartter syndrome?

As he looked closer, he found that, while all the children's mothers seemed to have had normal pregnancies and deliveries, all three infants had milk allergies and had therefore been placed on a soy-based formula.

Dr. Cordero soon discovered that there were five brands of soy-based formula on the market. All three of these children had consumed the same brand, Neo Mull Soy, manufactured by Syntex Corporation. He quickly learned that soy-based formulas represented only 3 percent of the formula market and that Neo Mull Soy was only 10-12 percent of the soy market. So Neo Mull Soy accounted for 0.3 percent of the formula market.

It would be surprising if all three infants, by chance alone, were using the same brand, but it could happen. So Dr. Cordero now took additional steps. He contacted the directors of the accredited pediatric nephrology training programs in the United States and asked whether they had seen cases of metabolic alkalosis in the previous year; if so, how many had they seen and had the affected children consumed infant formula? If they had, what brands were they using?

While anyone could conduct such a study, it is often difficult for a single scientist to focus beyond the immediate problem or to have the resources and the ability to enlarge the inquiry. A national program, such as at the CDC, has the opportunity to ask if this is part of a larger problem—national or even global—and the ability to then investigate beyond the local experience. Dr. Cordero, in a short period, was able to identify nineteen additional cases of recent metabolic alkalosis. Some programs would not identify the formula used, but when information was shared, it was consistent. They had used Neo Mull Soy.

A review of possible mechanisms led to the obvious question: Could these children have low consumption of chloride and potassium? If so, it made no logical sense that an infant formula would be deficient in essential electrolytes.

Cordero talked to the medical director of Syntex. The production of Neo Mull Soy seemed straightforward, and the company had even purchased the soy protein from the same source as other soy manufacturers. But there was one troubling point. Because of several episodes of bacterial contamination, Syntex had been delivering its product with a highly acidic pH to prevent additional bacterial contamination.

Even this finding was not a matter of early concern because the company indicated that it routinely measured electrolyte levels in its product and would have identified a problem in the product if the acidic pH had caused an electrolyte imbalance. In addition, Syntex had a repository of formula for each batch manufactured in the previous year so the company could re-test and recheck the results if that seemed to be needed.

On July 31, 1979, Dr. Cordero received a call from the Neo Mull Soy medical staff asking whether he could meet with them the next morning. They now related a problem previously unknown to them. Because of staffing problems that had occurred earlier, the company discovered a problem that had eluded all safeguards. The company review, which resulted from Dr. Cordero's inquiries, found that the company had been measuring sodium and potassium levels but not chloride levels. This had somehow been missed by everyone in the chain of command. In testing saved batches, they had found low or undetectable levels of chloride. They realized that they had made a mistake and would announce that they were recalling all formula nationwide.

Two Errors Provide Legal Protection

Fact is often stranger than fiction. Children clearly need adequate intake of chloride. If their diet is based on a purchased formula, that formula must contain chloride, or they will be in trouble, as this outbreak indicated. The company, by error, had not included chloride in the formula. But apparently, also by error, they had forgotten to list chloride in the ingredients. Therefore, according to the US Food and Drug Administration, they were not legally accountable. Two errors had occurred, but one of the errors resulted in legal protection.

Two of the mothers involved, Carol Laskin and Lynn Pilot, became active in a legislative solution so this could not happen again. The efforts resulted in Public Law 96-359, signed by President Carter on September 26, 1980.

Two points to close this chapter. The first is the absolute speed with which this investigation proceeded. The original problem was reported to the CDC on July 26, 1979. Within one week, the problem had been characterized, a national survey had been conducted, the biological explanation of low chloride intake was determined, a manufacturing error was discovered, and the product was removed from the market with an explanation of the findings distributed to the medical profession. A mere fourteen months after the first report, the president had signed a public law to prevent a similar event. This represented the CDC, the EIS, the Public Health Service, and the government at their best. It was a demonstration of why we need a strong government to do the things we cannot do ourselves. The usual answers to a strong government involve such matters as defense, regulations, roads, and rescue operations. In this case, it came down to vulnerable babies unprotected by the marketplace.

Some public health solutions require labor-intensive efforts, such as reducing smoking rates or reducing obesity. Others involve a combination of government decisions and behavioral changes, such as immunization programs. Other solutions are very efficient in requiring only government action, as in this case.

chapter 7

TOXIC SHOCK

Unexpected Deaths from an Improved Product

It was Monday, September 12, 2011. I was on a plane to Washington, DC, to speak at the tenth anniversary of the Measles Initiative. Many groups were involved in a global effort to interrupt measles transmission, an effort coordinated by the American Red Cross. Deaths had declined from more than 3 million per year to several hundred thousand. Amazing progress. The meeting would celebrate 1 billion measles immunizations administered to children around the world in the previous decade. The event was bound to be exciting.

On the plane I began reading the *New York Times* and suddenly gasped as I saw a picture of Bruce Dan. The article explained that he had died, at age 64, of complications following a bone marrow transplant for leukemia. The article recounted his life of adventure. He had received a bachelor's degree in aeronautics from MIT and a master's in biomedical engineering from Purdue. He then decided to go into medicine, getting his degree from Vanderbilt University. His wife described him as "a Renaissance man, always reinventing himself." He later spent time at the *Journal of the American Medical Association* and then became a medical news anchor.

Bruce's death took me by surprise, and I began to reminisce. Bruce had been part of the EIS while I was the CDC director. He, with two other physicians in that program, Kathy Shands and Art Reingold, plus a host of other workers at the CDC, had labored in 1980 to solve the mystery of women suddenly dying of a shock syndrome. The women would go from healthy to toxic to death in a matter of days. It was absolutely scary.

As soon as word got out that this condition existed, reports came in to the CDC by the dozens. The deaths were distributed throughout the country, and each had seemed to be a rarity at the place of report. When the reports were combined, however, it became clear that this was a national problem. Doctors were put on full alert, and the CDC investigators scrambled to make sense of it. The June 27, 1980, edition of the CDC's weekly newsletter reported on fifty-five cases of what was to become known as toxic shock syndrome (TSS) (1). Most patients were women, and most were between teenage years and age 50.

Senator Ted Kennedy held a hearing, asking the CDC to report on what it knew. Scientists frequently want some separation from politics, but it is not possible. Public health funding depends on appropriations from politicians. Therefore, when the CDC is called on to testify, the agency always has to agree. The problem is that answers are often unavailable early in an investigation; yet, the questioner will continue to probe. My general approach was to do the best preparation possible, bring a person with more knowledge on the subject, and then agree to get more information to provide for the record when we could not answer a question. I also learned over time to embrace the interest of politicians, to anticipate their knowledge needs before they asked, and to enlist them in the great adventure of public health. Every public health decision is ultimately based on a political decision.

For the TSS Senate hearing, I was accompanied by Dr. Shands and by Mrs. Robert Haley. Mrs. Haley had recovered from the syndrome and was asked to appear to report on what it was like to be a patient with this condition. Her husband, Robert Haley, worked at the CDC in hospital infections.

At one point, Senator Kennedy asked when we thought we would have an answer. Trying to combine optimism and realism and based on past investigations, I said, "I hope we have an answer by this fall." Dr. Shands told me later that she almost fell off her chair. They were still in the dark, and she did not see how they could unravel the mystery that soon.

But they did. The CDC, the Wisconsin State Department of Health and Social Services, and the Utah State Health Department undertook studies on the practices and products that might be in common use by the patients. While the reports included a wide spectrum of ages and included both male and female cases, the preponderance of female patients between the teen years and age 50 made it possible to narrow the focus to the menstrual cycle and then to tampons as a major risk factor, especially one tampon.

Calculating Risks

Late one Friday afternoon the investigation team reported on the risk inherent in using Rely tampons, manufactured by Procter & Gamble. Women did not make up all cases of toxic shock. When women were affected, not all cases involved the menstrual cycle. And if cases were related to the menstrual cycle, not all women affected had used Rely tampons. So it was a matter of figuring out the relative risk of various activities or products. If all cases had been in women who used Rely, then the answer would have been apparent and noncontroversial. Aware that the CDC had been criticized after the swine flu epidemic in 1976, for an appearance of basing decisions on scant evidence (see the "Swine Flu" section of chapter 9), three different and independent statistical groups at the CDC were convened to work over the weekend to analyze the statistics and render an opinion on the validity of the conclusion reached by the toxic shock investigative team.

On Monday morning, we gathered to hear each of the statistical groups report on its conclusions. I anticipated that all three would find the relationship to Rely tampons was firm. The three teams described their approaches, and two supported the conclusions with no qualifications. The third team expressed concern that calculations could be biased and therefore in error.

It was time to make a judgment. Based on all of the analysis, and aware of the concern of the third statistical team, we reached a tentative conclusion that Rely tampons were a risk factor. Certainty might be elusive but the health of the public required that we share our opinion. The CDC released its findings and on September 22, 1980, Procter & Gamble recalled Rely tampons voluntarily, notified consumers, and retrieved the product from the market.

The impact of the report was dramatic. In 1980, a total of 890 cases of TSS were reported, 812 (91 percent) were associated with menstruation, and 38 women with menstrual TSS died. In 1989, 61 cases of TSS were reported, and 45 (74 percent) were menstrual. There were no menstrual TSS deaths in 1988 and 1989.

Some scientists were concerned that the marked reduction was an artifact of the CDC's passive surveillance system, wherein cases are reported voluntarily. Therefore, a coalition of states developed a multistate active surveillance system, with investigators searching for cases. It found the same pattern. The rate of menstrual TSS declined from 6.2 cases per 100,000 women between 12 and 49 years of age in 1980 to 1 per 100,000 women later in the decade.

The precise mechanism by which Rely tampons increased the risk of TSS is unknown but may well have involved its heightened absorbency, which would require women to replace the tampons less often. This might have allowed time for bacterial growth and toxin production. But the result of taking them off the market was clear. The reporting of nonmenstrual toxic shock has remained fairly constant over the years.

Several lessons stand out. First, this was a life-and-death situation, and once again an EIS team, in a relatively short time period, took a chaotic situation and made sense of it. Second, the manufacturers had released a product that they felt was superior to other products on the market because of its high absorbency. An adverse outcome of low incidence is difficult to find in the relatively small numbers of subjects used in premarketing tests; therefore, postmarketing surveillance is essential to identify adverse effects of low incidence. A third lesson is the value of erring on the side of public health. The makers of Rely did not hesitate. Once the problem was identified, they quickly took the product off the market.

Fourth, once again public health was presented with a problem some-what different than that found in clinical medicine. In the latter, new findings may generate a great deal of excitement, but they are generally not accepted until repeated by another investigator. In public health, a second study is sometimes not possible. In the toxic shock incident, removing the product from the market was prudent but prevented a confirmatory study. The decision on reporting always has to be on the side of minimizing the chance for suffering and death—but with an awareness that an inaccurate report based on insufficient evidence could devastate an industry. Finally, the additional step of having three statistical groups reanalyze the findings was prudent.

chapter 8

SERENDIPITY AND UNEXPECTED PATHS

It was like reading a novel, when you can't read fast enough to satisfy your desire to know what is next. It was similar to the feeling I had when I read Albert Schweitzer's book *Out of My Life and Thought* (1) as a teenager. This time, it was the *New England Journal of Medicine*, and I was reading a commencement address given by physician Tom Weller to Harvard Medical School graduates (2). He was making the case for using skills and knowledge to benefit poor countries and even poor areas of rich countries with a plethora of problems and a paucity of resources and medical services. He was talking about the desire for more global equity in the area of health.

Tom Weller

I shared Weller's beliefs and assumed that I was being led away from the CDC to a new career in Africa. Little did I know that each step was actually and unexpectedly taking me back to the CDC.

Many years later, I would read lessons that a medical school classmate, Robert Eelkema, said that he had learned in life. The first one was "people in trouble do not need more trouble." Translated into a public health message, this means that when we retain our medical skills and knowledge only for ourselves and our immediate community, we allow people in trouble in countries that lack that knowledge to have more trouble.

I had no idea at the time, in my naiveté, that Weller was a Nobel laureate. When I got to know him, I learned that his Nobel Prize was for growing poliovirus in tissue culture. He demonstrated the old saying that chance rewards the prepared mind. He freely admitted that he had been trying for a different outcome. He had been attempting to grow the varicella (chickenpox) virus in a new broth, and, because he had several extra containers of broth leftover and did not wish to throw them out, he included poliovirus in the remaining broth containers on the spur of the moment. But he also replaced the nutrient material daily in the event that chickenpox virus was a slow-growing virus. The chickenpox virus did not grow. But to his surprise, the poliovirus did, and that breakthrough permitted Jonas Salk to grow virus and prepare a vaccine. Serendipity can be a powerful accelerator, as I was to learn later in smallpox eradication.

I applied and was accepted to spend a year, from 1964 to 1965, concentrating in the Department of Tropical Public Health, chaired by Weller, at the Harvard School of Public Health.

The CDC had offered me a position in its career development program, in which the CDC would pay for training programs of my choosing and I would then pay back a number of years of service at the agency. But I was eager to get to Nigeria, and so instead applied for a government scholarship, which allowed me to spend the year with Weller and go to Africa without an obligation to remain in the Public Health Service. (As it turned out, a war in Nigeria would return me to the CDC within a few years, which meant the agency got my employment but did not have to pay for the training.)

Being in Harvard's Department of Tropical Public Health was a wonderful experience. I got to be around a group who had dedicated their lives to the improvement of health in poor areas of the world. My faculty advisor, Frank Neva, was one of those rare people who could actually do research, pursue clinical medicine, teach, and be competent in all three endeavors.

But the faculty was only the beginning. Many of the students already had experience in developing countries. Charles Azu was a physician from Nigeria and would return to run a hospital with a public health perspective. Yemi Ademola was from a distinguished family in the former Western Region of Nigeria and had taken a year of leave from his position as head of prevention in the Nigerian Ministry of Health to get a master's in public health degree. Ademola was eager to teach me everything he could about his country and its health problems, and I was just as eager to learn. When a wrist injury left him unable to take notes, I had the chance to attempt to repay him for his kindness by providing him with carbon copies of my notes. He would later be very supportive of the work we were starting at a medical center in the Eastern Region of Nigeria and later, with our work with the CDC Smallpox Eradication/Measles Control Program in all of Nigeria. It was a tragedy and a great loss for Nigeria when he was murdered several years after graduation.

Fellow students Connie Conrad and Lyle Conrad had spent two years in Nigeria as part of the Peace Corps. These physicians not only retained an interest in global health but also continued to be colleagues, Lyle when we both worked at the CDC and Connie when we both worked at Emory University.

Formal classes were supplemented by spontaneous noontime debates on subjects I needed to understand but lacked the time to investigate, such as the efficacy of BCG (Bacille Calmette Guerin) or other vaccines not routinely used in the United States. A ten-day trip to the Public Health Service Leprosarium at Carville, Louisiana, provided training that would not be possible at Harvard. And, because this was the first time since fifth grade that I had not worked while going to school, I could also read for hours at a time—a luxury beyond belief.

During Weller's class, I made lifelong connections with faculty and students. I continued to see Frank Neva and Tom Weller over the next decades, and Tom often attended when I spoke in Boston. His wife said he took credit for any good thing I ever did and ignored the rest. She said he particularly liked to hear me when I would pull out his article that had contributed so much to my decision to go to Harvard. I would tell audiences that they had no idea of the ripple effects of what they say, do, or write. The year Tom retired I read his words at the commencement address given for the Harvard School of Public Health graduates. He got a standing ovation in the middle of my speech. A cycle had been completed.

Medical Work in Nigeria

Most of the Harvard graduates returned to their home countries or to positions with global health agencies or domestic public health agencies. Paula and I left Boston at the end of the school year, in June 1965, for a six-week course in St. Louis, Missouri, given by our new employers, the Lutheran Church-Missouri Synod (LCMS). The course taught culture, linguistics, and the requirements for employees of a church program in other countries. Surprisingly, there were few restrictions. My intent was to pursue community health and preventive medicine, and the church program was giving us the freedom to do that. All the synod asked for was a plan of action, after we had spent some time in Nigeria studying the problems, on how we hoped to improve the community health.

Most church-sponsored medical work at that time was clinically oriented. People in Africa, Asia, or other places are no different than people in the United States: they value medical care when it is needed. During illness or after injury, competent medical aid is a great comfort. So it is understandable that churches sponsoring medical work around the world invest in clinical approaches. But it is also true that it is less expensive and less disruptive to prevent disease and injury.

But LCMS had made the additional, bold decision to invest in disease and injury prevention. To make the situation even more unusual, LCMS was known for its conservative approach to religion and society. Even today, women are not given an equal status to men and cannot become ministers. Despite this gender bias and one of its well-known seminary professor's promoting racial bias at the time, this particular church body was willing to support work in prevention—work that, if optimally successful, would engender little gratitude, if any, on the part of those served and would therefore provide no benefit as a proselytizing tool. I found I could overlook a lot of things that made no sense for that kernel of goodwill that actually helped people.

While the organization sponsoring this prevention work was a surprise, an even greater one was that the genesis of this clear medical vision emanated from an unexpected person. Dr. Wolfgang Bulle had received his training in Germany during World War II. His training was interrupted by repeated terms of active duty. The atrocities of the war left him with what we would now undoubtedly diagnose as posttraumatic stress disorder. He always seemed to live his life at high speed to compensate for his involvement in that war.

Following surgical training, he spent ten years as a surgeon for LCMS in South India, a role for which he showed great creativity. For example, as a surgeon he needed a blood bank, but there was no possibility of developing one there. Instead, he identified a man who headed up a criminal network and made an arrangement. This man would send him dozens of people to have their blood typed. If Bulle needed blood from an O-positive donor, he would simply get a message to this man, telling him how many "volunteers" he needed and providing a list of the names of the people with that blood type. This walking blood bank was always available with no need for refrigeration facilities, outdated blood, and all the problems involved with blood banks. Bulle could reimburse the leader on the basis of the number of units drawn. The leader of the criminal network could keep part of the profits but also keep people eager to respond to the next call by providing donors with money.

Now, as head of LCMS's medical missionary program, Bulle sought efficiency, and prevention is efficient. The person who does not succumb to illness remains productive and consumes no medical resources. Surgeons who become interested in prevention are some of the most passionate workers in public health, and Bulle provided exceptional support to the work Paula and I were doing in Nigeria.

Paula and I experienced Africa by living in the village of Okpoma, in Ogoja Province in Eastern Nigeria. Although we did not have electricity, running water, or an indoor bathroom, life was easier for us than for the villagers, as we did not have to grow our own food, spend the day carrying water from distant locations, or secure firewood. Several nurses were already working in the area for the same church group, and they provided valuable insights into the problems of highest importance. Our plans for medical work matured as we experienced village life, observed the daily toil, and studied Yala, the local language. Our hopes were to expand child health services, especially immunization, diarrheal disease control, malaria control, water and sanitation programs, nutrition programs, and clinic services for all but especially children and pregnant women.

Jim and Gordon Hirabayashi

An unexpected boost to our efforts in Nigeria came from the chance meeting with anthropologist James Hirabayashi at a reception in Enugu, the capital of Eastern Nigeria. He was on leave from San Francisco State University for a one-year fellowship. Seeking interesting experiences, he asked whether he could visit our medical program to gather material on the culture of the Yala people with whom we were working. He was intrigued by what we were doing and asked to stay awhile. We provided him with an interpreter and transport, and he practiced his craft. During the day, he interviewed people living in Yala villages; at night, he typed up his notes and make entries on three-by-five cards, organizing his material by topic. Within weeks, he had discovered information about the culture unknown to LCMS missionaries who had been working in Ogoja Province for years. For example, there were social rules that governed who could marry into families. Illness was often understood in magical terms, and some illnesses actually resulted from curses that had been placed on individuals. Fatalism was at times the response to an illness if a person felt it was due to a curse. Hirabayashi also documented mechanisms that had developed to cope with death, illness, and unhappiness. For example, death was frequently followed by rituals that continued to celebrate a person even months and years later. Hirabayashi's work was intriguing and had direct relevance to a program hoping to improve health.

Unfortunately, the Nigerian (Biafran) Civil War interrupted his—and our—work.

A sidebar to this story: Back in Atlanta, some years later, I was reading about the internment of Japanese Americans when I encountered the legal case *Hirabayashi v. the United States*. Gordon Hirabayashi was a student at the University of Washington who resisted internment on the grounds that he could not be arrested without a reason. But he was arrested anyway and jailed in Seattle, while others were moved to an internment camp.

I called information in San Francisco and got a number for Jim Hirabayashi, my associate in Nigeria. He answered the phone, and I asked whether the legal case involved anyone in his family. It was his brother, Gordon, now a sociologist, who taught in Canada because he was not comfortable teaching in the United States. Jim said, "He happens to be visiting me tonight. Would you like to talk to him?" Gordon then related the story of how he resisted internment and was jailed. His case eventually went to the Supreme Court, where he lost unanimously. (A reminder that the Court is made up of fallible humans, and they have made some very un-supreme decisions.) After his loss at the Supreme Court, he learned that the government lacked the money to send him from jail in Seattle to the internment camp. So with great dignity, he hitchhiked and was admitted to the camp.

Gordon did not expect that the decision would ever be reversed. But years later, it was, and Gordon issued a statement about what a great country it is that can admit to that kind of mistake. In 2010, the University of Washington gave degrees to students who had been removed to the internment camps. I was pleased for Gordon—only to learn that he had Alzheimer's and was not aware of this second correction.

Gordon's final triumph came in 2012, when he was awarded the Presidential Medal of Freedom. Unfortunately, both Gordon and Jim died before the White House presentation.

If the Nigerian Civil War had been short, as I anticipated, we would have returned to renew our efforts to use a church medical program as a community health program. But the war became brutal and long, from July 1967 to early 1970. While I was able to work in the relief program during the war,

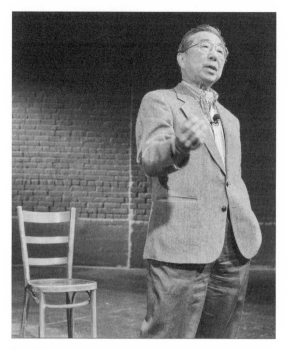

Dr. Gordon Hirabayashi. Courtesy of University of Alberta

my main job involved smallpox eradication, working from the CDC in Atlanta. When the war was over, I had become so obsessed with smallpox eradication that I could not return to Nigeria, at least at that time.

But the African experience was crucial in guiding the rest of my professional life. The needs of people living in poor countries could not be unlearned. The success with smallpox in Eastern Nigeria became a template for smallpox eradication in other countries. And the work of Jim Hirabayashi on the social determinants of health continued to resonate. The AIDS epidemic reinforced the need for anthropologists, sociologists, ethicists, theologians, and workers committed to social justice.

All of these experiences were totally unplanned by me. Beware of a life plan.

chapter 9

THE MYSTERIOUS DEATHS OF VETERANS

In 1976, the year of America's Bicentennial, Norman Cousins, the gifted political journalist and author, asked, in an editorial for the *Saturday Review*, "What is the greatest gift the United States has given the world in 200 years?" His answer: the demonstration that it is possible to plan a rational future.

Such a belief is indeed compelling. And it is one to which most public health practitioners subscribe. Optimistic by nature, they believe exerting some control over pathogens, diseases, even behavioral traits can have profound health benefits. Such a belief is the genesis of everything from vaccines to seat belt usage. Logic, carefulness, hard work, and mastery of one's field—these are the tools for planning.

But the Bicentennial year was to challenge that optimistic belief with a difficult, frustrating outbreak: Legionnaires' disease. This outbreak occurred at one of the worst times imaginable—on the heels of the nation's swine flu outbreak and vaccination program.

Swine Flu

A new influenza virus was isolated in January 1976 with many of the same characteristics as the flu virus that had killed 20 million people worldwide sixty years before. No specimens were available from that pandemic, but in the laboratory, the virus looked much as the experts expected the 1918 virus to look.

The CDC had found the 1976 influenza virus disturbing. It was a new influenza virus; it had demonstrated the ability to be transmitted from person to person during an outbreak at Fort Dix, New Jersey, and the population had no antibodies or evidence of immunity to this strain. All previous experience had shown that when these three things were documented, a pandemic would occur. Although it was possible that this could be the first time those elements came together without a pandemic, it certainly was not the way to bet.

CDC Director David Sencer held an emergency meeting of the Advisory Committee on Immunization Practices and other experts, on Saturday, February 14, 1976, which I attended. Participants agreed that a vaccine needed to be developed as fast as possible. Some disagreement arose on whether the vaccine, when manufactured, should be stored in refrigerators or in people. Phrased another way, should vaccine be stored until there was evidence of spread or should an immunization program be started in anticipation of the epidemic?

A case could be made for either side, but previous experience had raised serious doubts about the ability to respond in time to abort an outbreak if the vaccine were simply refrigerated. Once the vaccine is administered, it takes two weeks for an individual to develop immunity. A vaccine that requires the use of needles and syringes cannot be given as easily as a smallpox vaccine, for which untrained people can be trained in ten minutes on how to vaccinate. It would take some weeks to mount an adequate response with flu vaccine. Previous experience had also shown that a new strain of influenza virus could spread rapidly across the nation within weeks.

Dave Sencer realized the hazards of either decision. He listened to the arguments but did not call for a vote. He then made the decision to begin an immunization program, the Swine Flu Program. Later, to secure the necessary political support, a roomful of scientists, including Jonas Salk, inventor of the inactivated polio vaccine given by needle and syringe, and Albert Sabin, inventor of a live polio vaccine given by mouth, met in the Oval Office to make the case and to show their support for the idea when it was presented to President Gerald Ford.

But there were problems. Insurance companies would not insure vaccine producers for liability in the event the vaccine caused unforeseen morbidity or mortality, and manufacturers said they could not accept this risk without insurance. The government debated the issue, and publicity was intense. In July, with vaccine production in place, negotiations between the insurance companies and the manufacturers were breaking down.

A New Public Health Emergency

Now a second difficult outbreak hit. In Philadelphia, site of much of the Bicentennial celebration, people were already somewhat anxious. There was concern that terrorists might target the city in an attempt to disrupt the celebration. Extra security had been imposed.

On Wednesday, July 21, 1976, Legionnaires and family members from around Pennsylvania began to arrive in the city. They came first by the hundreds. Eventually, more than 4,000 arrived for the fifty-eighth convention of the American Legion. More than 600 of them would check into the Bellevue Stratford Hotel, headquarters for the convention.

The Bellevue Stratford had a rich history and a reputation for elegance. The hotel had served as the headquarters for the Republican Party at the 1936 National Convention and for both Democratic and Republican parties at the national conventions in 1948. It entertained royalty and presidents through decades of name changes and remodeling. It prided itself on being able to handle large, important gatherings.

But an organism, unknown to scientists at the time, had also checked into the Bellevue Stratford. That organism is now known as *Legionella pneumophila*. The public health community was destined to learn a great deal about this bacterium. It is found around the world. It is now easily isolated from ponds and streams, and it lives a symbiotic relationship with other organisms, often in one-celled organisms, such as amoebas. The genome has been determined; the eating habits and the methods of causing disease have been studied. It is inhaled directly into the small sacs in the lung, without being picked up by defense mechanisms in the bronchi, and it enters macrophages in the alveoli, or air sacs, of the lung.

The organism has probably been around as long as humans and has probably been in most, if not all, clinical laboratories, but it had never been recognized. Like the childhood fantasy of walking around invisible to others, this bacterium could go anyplace and not be recognized because no one had discovered how to stain it to make it visible nor how to prepare a food that it would consume and thus grow in the laboratory. The organism had also adapted to the modern technology of the twentieth century. It appears to enjoy the atmosphere of warm or hot water. It is especially fond of sediment and organisms found in air-conditioning and hot-water pipes.

While it does not spread from person to person, it is easily transmitted through aerosols, such as those formed when air leaves an air-conditioning unit or water leaves a showerhead. People have likely been getting pneumonia from this organism forever, and it has accounted for perhaps 3-4 percent of all pneumonias, but because it could not be isolated in the laboratory, the genesis of the pneumonia was listed as unknown or atypical.

None of this was known in 1976. But now a large number of people were about to be exposed to a particularly deadly aerosol, and the secret of this bacterium was to be revealed.

But it would not be disclosed without much time, agony, and hard work. A spectacular chapter was about to be played out in the history of public health, right under the gaze of William Penn's statue, who once said, "Healing the world is true religion."

As with previous conventions, the American Legion convention had hospitality suites, social events, and meetings—to conduct business, to honor veterans who had died in the last year, and to demonstrate the patriotism of this group brought together in defense of the country. Although it was not that different from many conventions, the veterans themselves were known to be heavy smokers and drinkers. Some have related these observations to veterans' war experiences, where cigarettes were distributed (indeed, cigarettes were included in the souvenir packages offered to attendees of the convention) and drinking became a stress reducer. The Bellevue Stratford actually ran out of ice on Thursday, the first day of the meeting, and the attendees began to bring in their own supplies of ice.

The beginning of an epidemic is not always sudden or dramatic. Who could imagine the illness of an air-conditioner repairman the day before the convention was a harbinger of what was to come? In a gathering of more than 4,000 people, it is expected that some will be sick at any given time. So when some attendees stayed in their rooms on Friday because they were not feeling well, it was not necessarily a cause for alarm. The only unusual part of the story was that Friday was a big day, with the annual parade in the afternoon and a dance at night. But some conventioneers were so ill that they actually went to bed that afternoon.

The closing session was held the next morning, and people began to drift home. Some began having respiratory symptoms and contacted their physicians. Rumors of influenza began to circulate, and suddenly Congress became concerned that this could be an outbreak of swine flu and quickly passed the Tort Claim Act, which would indemnify pharmaceutical companies against claims that might come from the Swine Flu Immunization

Program. This swift action allowed the Swine Flu Immunization Program to proceed . . . but this was not swine flu.

Soon information was coming back from clinics and hospitals to local and state health authorities of conventioneers who developed pneumonia after returning home from the convention. The CDC officially became involved on Monday, August 2, when Bob Craven, an EIS officer with the Respiratory and Special Pathogens Branch, received a call from a nurse at the Veterans Administration Hospital in Philadelphia, who reported two cases of pneumonia in attendees of the convention; one of the patients had died.

A flurry of phone calls throughout the day soon revealed eighteen known deaths of attendees, most from pneumonia, and an additional seventy-one case-patients in hospitals throughout Pennsylvania. That is an unusual number of deaths in a short period. The immediate thought that this could be due to influenza was understandable.

Fraser in Charge

The subsequent investigation was to be one of the largest ever undertaken by the CDC. It was headed by Dr. David Fraser, an intense, clear-thinking epidemiologist who reveled in the complex and mysterious world of newly discovered pathogens. His team would demonstrate the value of the CDC's history of training a group that might be needed if the country ever faced bioterrorism. Some were former members of the EIS, including Dr. Bob Sharrar, now chief of communicable disease in Philadelphia. Some were current EIS officers who would go on to other public health positions in the future, including Dr. Steve Thacker, who later became head of the program to train these "disease detectives," and Dr. David Heymann, who would later head up the communicable disease programs of the WHO. They were only a few of the dozens of CDC epidemiologists assigned to Fraser, supplementing dozens of state employees. Scores of others were involved in testing specimens from patients and the environment and supporting the huge logistic needs of the investigators.

The large team instituted intense surveillance, contacting hospitals and clinics. They sought help on cases by establishing a hotline to immediately provide information to the public. As the cases and deaths mounted, attempts were made to culture an organism, and specimens were collected for testing for toxic agents.

In a surprising development, tests for influenza were negative, as were cultures for known causes of pneumonia. By noon of August 3, a case definition had been developed and approximately 100 persons fit the category. An EIS officer visited each person, a chart review and physical exam were completed, and cases were excluded or included based on this review. By the evening of August 5, the list included 140 persons.

There was no clue of an etiological agent. However, an important finding had been established—there had been no secondary spread from these patients, a fact that provided some reassurance to the public. This was important because family members were understandably concerned that they might be next, and some people were shunning those who had attended the convention. The lack of an influenza virus in cultures and of secondary spread was sufficient to eliminate influenza as a possible cause.

Among attendees, visiting the Bellevue Stratford Hotel was strongly associated with illness. Although only about 15 percent of the attendees had actually stayed at this hotel, many had visited it for the meetings.

Because thousands of phone calls came in to the CDC investigators, a triage system was developed so that EIS officers could concentrate on what investigators hoped would be the most productive leads. First, to characterize the illness, each patient was contacted for follow-up information. While incubation periods varied, and some attendees were sick by the end of the convention on July 24, the average person's symptoms developed six days after arrival at the convention. Few cases developed after August 1. The illness was characterized by fever and cough, severe enough that 80 percent of patients were hospitalized. Fevers over 104°F, rapid pulse, and rapid breathing were more common in those who died.

But still no agent could be identified. Organic and inorganic toxic agents were also sought in environmental samples and tissue samples at autopsy. Every test ended in frustration.

The analysis suggested higher attack rates in persons who actually stayed at the Bellevue Stratford than those who did not. In addition, persons who developed symptoms but had not stayed at the hotel were found to have spent more time at the hotel for meetings than did those who did not get sick. Finally, the highest rates of illness seemed to be related to time spent in the hotel's lobby. The lack of illness in hotel employees was noted, but the employees tended to be much younger than the guests, so they did not provide a true comparison group. These were all good clues, but they did not add up to an answer.

The investigation continued through the fall, the team always hoping for new information that would explain what was not making sense. It seemed clear to the investigators that this was an infectious agent, but the science was failing them.

No investigation is complete without red herrings, and while public health investigations don't require such problems, sometimes they appear. The red herring came from a respected scientist, F. William Sunderman. Dr. Sunderman was exceptional in many ways. He was a first-class pathologist, musician, globalist (and survivor, living to the age of 104), as well as a world authority on the toxic effects of nickel carbonyl. He suggested that the epidemic was due to nickel carbonyl. CDC-gathered specimens were not adequate for the analysis required, and the early autopsy specimens supported the theory. It was then discovered that the pathologists had gathered the specimens by using metal instruments and that they were the possible sources of the nickel. Sunderman himself did the retesting and found the evidence wanting. The theory was discarded, and the investigation continued.

Cyril Wecht, coroner of Allegheny County, Pennsylvania, was politically ambitious, outspoken, controversial, and a magnet for journalists. He was publicly critical about what he thought was being done wrong in the Legionnaires' disease investigation, and, consequently, both Pennsylvania and the CDC health officials were placed on the defensive. Outspoken critics can be helpful in setting priorities and making decisions. If they are on your team, it is useful to enlist them in exploring their theories and making midcourse corrections when appropriate. But if they aren't on your team and instead act as outside commentators, with no responsibility to test their suggestions, they require an inordinate amount of energy and time just to answer their charges. It is far easier to be disruptive than helpful.

Congress Weighs In

But the biggest nemesis was congressman John M. Murphy, chair of the congressional Subcommittee on Consumer Protection and Finance. Murphy was accomplished and powerful. Born on Staten Island, he had attended Amherst College and West Point. During his twelve years of military service, he was awarded the Distinguished Service Cross and the Bronze Star. He had demonstrated his abilities, but he had also become addicted to the spotlight.

Murphy was determined to have a hearing to show the CDC's incompetence. The press had been harsh about the CDC's inability to find a cause for the outbreak, and media attention fed Murphy's approach. The CDC had quickly ruled out dozens of outbreak possibilities, an astounding accomplishment from a scientific perspective. But it didn't make up for its failure to find the cause. Congressman Murphy now scheduled two days of hearings in Philadelphia to hammer home the incompetence of the CDC. Dave Fraser would be the major witness at these hearings, but he was joined by Drs. Sencer and Joseph Boutwell, deputy director of the Bureau of Laboratories at the CDC. Dave Sencer was determined to take the heat by actually reading the opening statement on behalf of all three witnesses.

Congressmen generate headlines, and so the anticipation of hearings in Philadelphia again increased the negative stories about the CDC's inability to solve the outbreak. To make matters worse, Murphy circulated a memo to his committee that indicated that he would label the investigation "a fiasco." The memo was leaked to Jack Anderson. Anderson was a journalist, radio and TV personality, and a heavyweight in investigative reporting circles. He was unafraid of powerful people and was known for revealing information on J. Edgar Hoover (even going through Hoover's garbage cans). He was bold in fighting battles but not always right. For example, he sided with Senator Joseph McCarthy in his hunt for communists until the evidence against McCarthy became overwhelming. Anderson published an article on Legionnaires' disease that denigrated the CDC and its experts as people who had a high regard for themselves—one not shared by the rest of the scientific community. This was going to be a hostile hearing.

On Tuesday, November 23, Congressman Murphy opened the hearing and did not disappoint those looking to find fault. His opening statement was belittling to those who had worked hard for four months to entertain every possibility, seek out every clue, and review every finding. He said, "CDC's apparent failure to consider all possible causes from the very beginning, no matter what their expectations led them to believe, is questionable." He believed a toxin was the cause of Legionnaires' disease and that the CDC was so focused on an infectious cause that it had failed to see the big picture.

The day went on with a variety of witnesses. The CDC's statement was put off until the next morning. At that time, Dave Sencer read a careful statement that reviewed what had been found and suggested that this was not a human failure but rather a reflection of where the science was at this time.

The questions that followed the opening statement were not so much questions as continuing attacks on the witnesses. Reason was brushed aside, and the three CDC witnesses experienced what many have learned: the power of science is often neutralized by the power of power.

It was a moment of low morale for the CDC. The Legionnaires' outbreak was a frustrating example of coming up short. There had been outbreaks in the past that were not solved. But usually the reason was understandable. A delay may have made it impossible to get proper samples—or none may have been available (a frequent occurrence in foodborne outbreaks). Sometimes, as in an outbreak of respiratory problems in Pontiac, Michigan, the samples seemed adequate, but no organism was identified. But even with organisms never before seen, as with Lassa fever, green monkey disease, or Ebola, modern laboratory techniques had risen to the occasion and identified, for the first time, an organism not previously known.

The outbreak of Legionnaires' disease provided sufficient clinical patients, compulsive investigators, and samples of almost everything—but no solution. It was more than frustrating. It was demoralizing. Highly trained investigators were rendered impotent.

A month after the congressional hearing, David Fraser finished his report and in seventy-nine pages summarized what had been found. The summary of those seventy-nine pages is muted, and it requires some insight to understand the hard work; the countless hours; the political, scientific, and social barriers faced; and the unhappiness and frustration of not being able to find the cause of this outbreak:

SUMMARY—An outbreak of 180 cases of febrile respiratory illness with 29 deaths occurred in Philadelphia in July and August 1976. One hundred forty-nine of the cases were in persons who had attended an American Legion Convention held at Hotel A and the remainder had all entered the hotel. Results of the epidemiologic investigation indicated that continuing common-source transmission occurred during the convention, and that age, delegate status at the convention, and spending time in Hotel A were determined to be risk factors for illness. No mode, place, or vehicle of transmission could be incriminated with certainty. The outbreak terminated spontaneously, and no spread to the City of Philadelphia was found. (Unpublished CDC communication)

Resolution

The story was not over. Restless scientists at the CDC continued to second-guess themselves. Joe McDade, an expert on *Rickettsia* organisms, attended a party on the evening of December 28 of that year, but he was troubled and returned to his lab to search once again through the slides he had prepared from samples submitted months earlier from the Philadelphia outbreak. He later described the effort as similar to searching for a contact lens on a basketball floor by oneself.

He had been asked to rule out Q fever and had inoculated guinea pigs with material from patients who had died. The guinea pigs died, but no organisms could be found in the guinea pig samples. He *had* seen occasional inclusions in scavenger cells that looked like bacteria, but they seemed insignificant because if they had caused disease the sample would have been swarming with the bacteria.

This night, however, he noticed something that excited him. He saw a number of bacteria inside a white cell. The next day, he and his team started from scratch. Because the bacteria were not showing up with the usual staining techniques, the lab team tried new ways of staining and new ways of growing the organism.

Within two weeks, McDade, his mentor Dr. Charlie Shepard, and their staffs had located the new organism, figured out how to make it grow, and found a way of staining it so that it could be seen under the microscope. Then they had shown that survivors of the Pennsylvania outbreak had antibodies to this exact organism.

The scientists determined that the newly named *Legionella* organisms do not grow under typical laboratory conditions. They require a specialized diet of cysteine and iron, low sodium, and activated charcoal. They also thrive in higher temperatures than most bacteria.

The team kept these findings absolutely quiet until they were sure of their results. Even then they had reservations. But it was time to tell.

Roslyn "Robbie" Robinson, director of the CDC Laboratories, asked for an appointment with Dave Sencer. Robinson brought with him Walt Dowdle, head of virology; Dr. Shepard, a world-renowned leprologist; and Dr. McDade, a rickettsiologist, to the meeting with the CDC's director. After some hemming and hawing, as Sencer later reported it, Robbie said, "I guess we should tell you that Shep and Joe have isolated the organism that causes Legionnaires' disease."

"After a minute of stunned silence," Sencer said, "they explained that the two had been using old microbiological techniques to see if they could recover an organism, and they had. I called Dave Fraser to come down along with Don Berreth [director of the CDC's Office of Information] . . . Shep said they wanted to take the weekend to redo the isolation in a room where they had not been working to rule out any possibility of contamination."

The scientists confirmed the findings over the weekend, and Berreth developed a plan for a special edition of the *Morbidity and Mortality Weekly Report* (*MMWR*) to be released on Tuesday, January 18, 1977. The presses were running that day when Sencer said, "Shep came literally running into my office, to tell me that he had retrieved sera from the serum bank of two earlier unresolved outbreaks of pneumonia and they were positive for the identical organism. The presses stopped, the corrections were made, and from then on it moved like clockwork."

That Tuesday, January 18, there was also a conference call of health officers around the country, and every CDC worker involved in any way with the investigation was on the call. This was followed by a CDC press conference, at which Sencer announced to gathering journalists that the cause of Legionnaires' disease was now known. It was a time to rejoice over the ability of science to unravel yet another complex problem.

Before the press conference, Sencer contacted his superiors in Washington, DC, so that they would not be surprised by the announcement. He even had the courtesy to call Congressman Murphy to say that, after an exhausting series of tests, McDade and Shepard were confident that they understood the cause of the Philadelphia outbreak. The congressman responded, "Well, it's about time."

Three days later, Congressman Murphy issued a newsletter with the banner headline: "CONGRESSMAN MURPHY CONFIRMS THE CAUSE OF LEGIONNAIRES DISEASE."*

*Less than four years later, in December 1980, the press reported that Congressman Frank Thompson Jr. and Congressman John M. Murphy had been found guilty in the FBI undercover Abscam probe—Thompson for bribery and conspiracy and Murphy for receiving an unlawful gratuity, conflict of interest, and conspiracy.

chapter 10

AN UNEXPECTED RETURN TO THE CDC

I flash back to 1966. As Paula and I became more comfortable in our new culture as medical missionaries in Nigeria, opportunities for health improvements began to appear. Living in a village allowed us to understand the rhythm of daily life, to understand the risks that villagers confronted daily, and to think about solutions that might be reasonable for that context.

We were, in a sense, living within a bubble, observing the village. Although we did not have electricity, running water, or an indoor bathroom, we coped. During the rainy season, the water supply was adequate. Roof water was caught in a gutter to fill a fifty-five-gallon drum. We dipped water from the drum for baths into a metal tub in the bedroom. We boiled water for drinking. Without electricity, we used a kerosene stove and a kerosene refrigerator to preserve food and to cool boiled water used for drinking and cooking.

During the dry season, we hired a young man to carry water in two five-gallon tins (about eighty pounds) on the back of his bicycle. These he would empty into the fifty-five-gallon drum. As the dry season progressed, the distance traveled to find water increased. By the end of the dry season, two trips a day would be the norm, and water conservation became important.

Screened windows, bed nets, and chloroquine as a malaria prophylactic protected us from the disease that plagued the rest of the village. Bouts of fever were common for both children and adults. A certain degree of immunity to malaria developed in villagers. But this immunity was not absolute.

And while it modified the intensity of each bout with malaria, the illness was still debilitating, at best, with deaths common in children and in pregnant women. Malaria prophylaxis for those two groups became very important. Immunizations provided protection against other diseases, and wearing shoes or sandals protected against hookworm.

It became clear to Paula and me that two factors, not shared by villagers, provided us protection for our own child. The first was knowledge that we had acquired. This was potentially transferable to all persons in the village. The other factor was money. If we had been limited to a dollar a day per person, as they were, it would have been enough for food and shelter, but it would have left nothing for vaccines, screens, or the wood required to boil water. Vaccinating the village children, treating malaria, and providing safe water, sanitation, and dietary improvements were all basic needs. But providing them would require ingenuity plus outside resources to launch such projects.

Serendipity once again intervened. The CDC asked me to be a short-term consultant as it initiated the Smallpox Eradication Program in West and Central Africa, part of a global effort to eradicate the disease. Henry Gelfand, an epidemiologist with the smallpox program, was sent to Enugu to talk to me about the possibility. He made it clear that he did not think this was a good idea, but he was carrying out orders. He did not think the CDC needed part-time consultants. I, however, saw this as a great opportunity to become acquainted with the Nigerian public health system, which held promise for our future work. Accepting the request led to a visit back to the CDC in the summer of 1966 to participate in the training program for forty-three CDC personnel about to be assigned to twenty countries in West and Central Africa.

Smallpox in Eastern Nigeria

While we were back in the United States, our second son, Michael, was born in Walla Walla, Washington, the home of my parents. Paula and I and our two boys then prepared for our return to Nigeria. I went ahead to set up a flat for the next year in Enugu. Suddenly, we had running water and electricity. Lawrence Atutu Ochelebe, who had worked with us in the village and then at the medical compound, now joined me in Enugu to establish the flat. (Lawrence was perceptive and loyal. Some months later, he told me that he could not be sure but he thought that a neighbor had managed to tie into our electric line, and we were therefore paying their electricity bill. That night he turned off our main electrical circuit while I watched to see what would happen at the neighbor's flat. Indeed, the neighbor's flat went black—as did half a city block!)

Soon Paula arrived with David and Michael, and we settled in. Next, the Thompsons arrived. David Thompson was a physician, trained in pediatrics, and Joan Thompson was a nurse. A second CDC assignee, public health advisor Paul Lichfield, arrived with his wife, Mary.

We entered into six months of hard work. It started with an outbreak investigated on December 4, 1966, the month before the program was to officially start. We had not yet received our major supplies and therefore could not do mass vaccinating in the area as we would ordinarily have done. We were reduced to vaccinating only those people we felt were at immediate risk of exposure—family members, village neighbors, and those who had contacted the persons with smallpox.

The missionaries had nightly radio contact, and we were able to use that means of communication to provide geographic assignments; the next day, the missionaries could send people to every village in their assigned area to find smallpox cases. Within twenty-four hours, we knew which villages already had smallpox, which enabled us to be precise in our vaccination efforts. The outbreak stopped quickly, and we received permission from the medical authorities in Eastern Nigeria to expand the idea of precision vaccination (later called surveillance/containment), rather than mass vaccination, to stop smallpox. But we also needed to institute a program to immunize children from 6 months to 6 years of age for measles. That required a mass approach. We were able to combine the two needs by identifying smallpox outbreaks and, in those areas, attacking smallpox quickly through selective vaccinations, and at the same time, we launched the mass vaccination program for both measles and smallpox in the geographic areas involved. The abrupt movement of teams to Enugu, cited later in the chapter, provides an example of rapid changes in plans to protect against smallpox while still protecting children from measles.

With experience, surveillance improved. To the best of our knowledge, we detected every smallpox outbreak in Eastern Nigeria within the first six months of the campaign. Some were small, a handful of cases, but some were large. One outbreak, in Abakaliki Province, some forty miles from Enugu, included more than 1,000 cases. Temporary shelters were constructed outside of towns and villages, and persons who had previously had smallpox delivered food and provided the interface with those so quarantined.

As recounted in *House on Fire* (1), we were successful in getting supplies even when the federal government of Nigeria halted shipments to the region. We were working on the last known outbreak in the Eastern Region when we were asked to attend a meeting, in Accra, Ghana, of people assigned from the CDC throughout the twenty-country area. What would later be known as the Nigerian Civil War was building to a flash point, but a check with the American Consulate in Enugu was reassuring: they expected fighting would be delayed for some months as both the federal government and the Biafra military had to recruit and train soldiers as well as purchase supplies. It seemed reasonable to leave for a few days for the meeting in Ghana and then return to continue the program.

Our wives and children had been evacuated two months earlier in anticipation of fighting, but those of us remaining were not overly concerned about leaving, as the consulate thought there would be sufficient warnings that would allow us time to leave before the fighting broke out. However, the large number of roadblocks constituted a barrier to efficient travel, and at times, the stops could be unnerving. Often the people checking vehicles would be teenagers, fueled by beer and wielding AK-47s. The combination was potentially explosive and required a cool, respectful approach on our part.

For the Accra meeting, we prepared materials on our experiences to demonstrate how we had implemented surveillance and containment activities throughout the region. Maps highlighting the locations of outbreaks and vaccination efforts were copied for distribution. The mixture of mass vaccination and surveillance/containment we were practicing was a departure from the instructions given in the training program at the CDC. Indeed, the field manual was clear in warning against being distracted by smallpox outbreaks lest those diversions detract from the orderly plan of mass vaccinations. Jumping from outbreak to outbreak did not appear orderly. Therefore, we attempted to document everything to explain the deviation from the plan.

For example, a Saturday morning meeting in our smallpox headquarters in Enugu had been interrupted by the news that smallpox patients had been admitted to the Enugu General Hospital. We immediately verified the diagnosis and then changed our intended activities for the next week. This seemed anything but orderly. We decided to move vaccination teams both to Enugu and to the area where the smallpox patients had been discovered. We used the rest of the weekend to plot sites for vaccination teams on Monday and developed a schedule for when they would move from site to site. As we vaccinated against smallpox, we also protected all children under age 6 from measles, combining mass vaccination with surveillance/containment.

It was while finding vaccination sites and marking them on my enlarged map of Enugu that I was arrested and spent the remainder of Saturday being questioned by the police. Prison in Nigeria is not a sought-after experience. But interestingly, my concern at the moment was for the time being lost for planning Monday's activities. I assumed I would be released. From their perspective, with the possibility of civil war discussed daily in the newspaper, having an outsider putting marks on maps was threatening. It was late in the afternoon before they were able to locate the medical person in charge of smallpox eradication in Eastern Nigeria. He came to the police station and was able to secure my release.

The outbreak was contained, as were all other known outbreaks, and we left for the Accra meeting with our teams working on the last known outbreak. We expected to return, document the absence of smallpox in all of Eastern Nigeria, and continue with the mass vaccination program that would protect from smallpox importations and would provide measles protection to children.

Getting to the meeting required taking a small boat across the Niger River and having our passports stamped on both the Biafra side and then the Nigerian side. We hired a taxi to take us to Lagos and then on to Accra. We had been there only a few days when we heard that fighting had broken out on the Biafra borders and that we would not be able to reenter Eastern Nigeria.

Civil War

The civil war in Nigeria brought an abrupt change in many plans. Since I could not return to Enugu, I tried working in Northern Nigeria, expecting that it would be a short period of fighting, and one side or the other would quickly back down. I was totally mistaken about the length of the fighting, which went on until early 1970, over two and a half years of agonizing fighting and civilian starvation.

I was asked by the Nigerian national smallpox program to evaluate what was happening in Sokoto Province. I soon departed in one of the program's Dodge trucks with camping equipment and information on where I would find the teams. On the first night in the field, I had just completed erecting a tent and was cooking dinner when a police vehicle appeared. The policeman came up to me and handed me a piece of paper with my name on it. "Is this you?" he asked. I said it was, and he said, "You are under arrest." He would give me no information regarding the charges or what was wrong.

I was put in the back of the police vehicle with armed guards on each side. We headed back for Kaduna.

On the way, the group decided to stop at a rest house for beer. They left me sitting alone in the back of the vehicle. That is when I noticed there was a pistol on the front seat. Was this a trap? I decided not to move, and on their return, they showed no surprise at finding me still sitting there. This was much more nerve-racking than the arrest in Enugu. The reason for the arrest was not clear, and I was sitting between beer-drinking armed guards, barreling down an African highway . . . a perfect storm of risk factors.

In Kaduna, I was questioned about the purpose of my trip and put under house arrest. It soon became clear that the real problem was that I had been working in the Eastern Region, now fighting Nigeria as Biafra. What information was I trying to get, and did I still have contacts in Biafra? The rest of Nigeria was now at war with the Eastern Region and therefore anyone who had worked in the Eastern Region was regarded with suspicion. Questioning continued the next day and to my surprise included questions on the names of family members and their locations. The decision was made that I could be released, but only if I left Nigeria. This I did, but I was able to travel back to Nigeria many times over the next few years without this arrest coming to light.

When I returned to Atlanta in the fall of 1967, the CDC offered to put me on contract until I could return to the medical center in Yahe, Nigeria, to continue my work with the church health program. I accepted and worked for Dr. Don Millar on smallpox eradication. Under Don's direction, physician Mike Lane, public health advisor Jim Hicks, and I divided responsibilities for overseeing the CDC program; my area included Nigeria, Ghana, Liberia, and The Gambia.

One of my obsessions was to expand the idea of surveillance/containment to other areas of West Africa and to figure out how best to implement that approach. Program agreements had been signed with each country. A basic tenet of these agreements was that there would be an attack phase of mass vaccination to be completed in three years. All ages would be vaccinated against smallpox and children under 6 against measles. A paper by Henry Gelfand and D. A. Henderson, who had been assigned from the CDC to head up the WHO program in Geneva, had indicated that the mass vaccination cycle might be followed by a second mass vaccination campaign, if indicated. In each country, an attempt would be made to improve the reporting system—to understand the size of the smallpox problem and its distribution but also to serve as the basis for concentrating resources to implement containment of outbreaks as the mass campaign brought down the incidence of smallpox.

Complicating the development of a new smallpox strategy was, of course, the second component of the program, measles control. Measles was a horrendous disease in West and Central Africa, feared by parents and health officers. At the time the smallpox/measles program started, the measles virus was the single most lethal agent in the world. It accounted for at least 3 million deaths a year; some thought the numbers were even higher. It killed more people than tuberculosis. Any change in the smallpox approach had to do justice to measles control. Africa was correct in wanting a program for measles. The United States Agency for International Development (USAID) also was interested and valued this part of the program above smallpox. Indeed, for the entire length of the program, the CDC called the program the Smallpox Eradication/Measles Control Program; USAID called it the Measles Control/Smallpox Eradication Program.

The name was not the important thing. The important thing was that the two agencies had so much trouble working together on common objectives. The lack of trust seemed unbridgeable. The CDC was concerned that USAID was trying to use the program for political purposes, while USAID thought the CDC was diverting resources from the program to other CDC activities.

On one occasion, a USAID employee spent a week at the CDC to understand the program and to improve coordination between the two agencies. When I invited him home for dinner on Monday night of that week, it became apparent that he had a drinking problem. He became convinced of my sincerity over dinner and that, combined with the loss of his inhibitions, led him to ask, "Do you have any idea why I am really here?" I did not.

"I have been asked to find if you are diverting USAID funds to other areas of CDC," he said. He then described himself as the right person to do this since as USAID country director in a South American country, he had kept two sets of books in order to divert funds. This incident was symptomatic of the problems we encountered to the very end of the program.

But the immediate difficulty was how to combine the needs of the measles program, which required a mass vaccination program in every geographic area, with the flexibility required for smallpox surveillance/containment, which required the ability to concentrate on the areas with smallpox outbreaks. The solutions were found in various ways. In some countries, such as Dahomey (now Benin), a separate group of twelve health workers on motorcycles concentrated on smallpox outbreaks, while the rest of the staff worked on a smallpox/measles mass vaccination program. In other countries, smallpox workers were diverted as needed for outbreak control but worked also on mass programs. In all countries, the areas of smallpox were circumscribed; therefore, they were not spread evenly throughout the country. This meant that smallpox vaccination numbers continued to climb because of mass vaccination, even if most of the vaccinations were conducted in areas where there was no smallpox. Those vaccinations had no impact on the disease. This was confusing to those not familiar with the program, and at least one statistician at Yale, looking at total numbers of vaccinations, rather than the geographic distribution of those vaccinations, later interpreted the reduction of smallpox to mass vaccination rather than to targeted activities.

In most areas, the experiences of early adopters, that is, those who focused on containment of all smallpox outbreaks, helped to improve on smallpox-eradication activities. For example, it became clear that the smallpox virus had adapted to thousands of years of evolution. It did the virus little good to spread rapidly, exhausting susceptible people in a single generation. Rather, it spread in a slow and deliberate fashion through a household and through a village. This allowed the virus to linger for an extended period, increasing the chance of exposing a visitor, who could take the virus elsewhere. This unique pattern of smallpox provided the opportunity to identify an outbreak and break chains of transmission.

Strike at the Right Moment

It was also clear that smallpox was a seasonal disease and would decrease during the rainy season when human contact and activities decreased because of the difficulty of transportation. (There was also perhaps an inhibiting effect of high humidity on the transmissibility of the virus during the rainy season.) These were the times when mass vaccination was most difficult. However, it was possible to increase the efficiency of the program by increasing the smallpox efforts at that time. Small teams on bicycles or walking could still access remote areas. We emphasized that a chain of transmission broken during this low period of transmission would prevent hundreds of cases over the next year, while a chain of transmission broken during high transmission, while useful, would prevent far fewer new cases over the next year. Approached in this manner, it becomes clear that as difficult as it was to work in the rainy season, a small number of workers could be far more efficient than the usual approach. It is a lesson for all of public health. While the best decisions are based on the best science, the best results are based on the best management, and this was a good management practice. In various ways, it was possible to combine surveillance/containment directed at smallpox while also doing mass vaccination for both diseases.

With EIS officers taking the lead, we studied every country in the African program. Some countries' programs, such as Sierra Leone's, under the leadership of Don Hopkins, emphasized surveillance/containment from the beginning and made dramatic progress.

Smallpox Eliminated from West Africa

The original plan was to eradicate smallpox in the twenty countries in five years. It went even faster than planned. The last case in the twenty-country area was reported from Nigeria in May 1970, three years and five months after the program began. The objective was reached a year and a half early and under budget.

The last sentence hides an incredible amount of work by dozens of CDC people stationed in Africa, dozens remaining in Atlanta, thousands of Africans, and an unseen coalition who produced vaccines and supplies, shipped them, stored them, and got them to the right place at the right time. The complexity of that web and the chain of events that finally gets a vaccine into a person are beyond comprehension. No wonder Harland Cleveland once characterized global health workers as people with unwarranted optimism.

Just as significant for the local population was the rapid reduction in measles. Children went from a 7 percent risk of dying from this disease to an environment that increased their chances of reaching adulthood. It was a great and optimistic time. Unfortunately, USAID changed its priorities when a new person became the administrator for the program, and the measles program was brought to an abrupt end—before ministries of health could institutionalize measles immunization in their budgets and ministry programs. Years later, USAID, to its credit, again funded measles programs in Africa, but continuity was lost, and Africans suffered between the two efforts.

USAID has done such important work over the decades, but the fact that it is embedded in the State Department is a flaw because political concerns will always factor into its selection of priorities. When there is a health problem in the United States, the chain of command is clear, and, ultimately, the secretary of the Department of Health and Human Services (HHS) is held responsible. By contrast, a health problem outside our borders leads to confusion. It takes time to determine whether the problem will be handled by the secretary of HHS, USAID, the secretary of state, the National Security Agency, an ambassador, the Red Cross, or all of them. Having all health problems centralized as the responsibility of one person, the secretary of HHS, would reduce this confusion. This change would also ensure that the health priorities of US citizens would benefit from the perspective of global events and that global decisions would benefit from knowledge of domestic approaches. The Ebola outbreak of 2014 again demonstrates the problems inherent in not having a single person, the secretary of HHS, charged with the responsibility of coordinating the US response.

chapter 11

DISASTER RELIEF

Again, the unexpected. As I have mentioned, it is one of the reasons that I advise students against developing a life plan. The world changes so fast that there is no way to predict what opportunities—or disasters—will appear.

Civil war continued to rage in Nigeria, and both sides found sources of arms that prolonged the fighting. The rebels were surrounded, so they developed a system of dangerous night flights into the Biafra enclave: planes turned on their lights to land on a road only at the last moment to reduce the chance of being bombed by Nigerian planes.

The International Committee of the Red Cross

Soon stories of starvation were reported from the "Republic of Biafra." Ordinarily, the League of the Red Cross responds to such conditions. The League was established in 1919 to represent National Red Cross societies around the world. However, since there was now a Nigerian Red Cross and a Biafran Red Cross, the League could not be a neutral representative. In cases such as this, the International Committee of the Red Cross (ICRC) becomes responsible. The two groups (the League and the ICRC) are often confused, especially because both have headquarters in Geneva, Switzerland. But

ICRC is much older, dating to 1863, and it is actually a private organization, established by Swiss citizens. It represents victims of war and has a stellar reputation, which has led to Nobel Prizes on three occasions.

Wolfgang Bulle had been appointed field coordinator in Nigeria by the ICRC. In late summer 1968, I received a telegram asking whether I would join Wolf as deputy field coordinator of relief activities in Nigeria. I showed the telegram to Don Millar, my supervisor. Strongly irritated, he told me I would have to decide whether I was still working for the mission or whether I was now working for the CDC. With that he left the room.

I was disturbed throughout the day as I weighed the request, knowing he was correct. To complicate the situation, our son Michael had just recovered from croup, which had required hospitalization. He was frightened, and when the doctors made rounds they found that Paula had actually climbed into his oxygen tent to hold him. He required minor surgery to insert a tube into his trachea to allow him to breathe. Seeing him breathing easily again was such a relief, but the poignant memory of him, unable to speak, lying in bed with tears rolling down his cheeks continued to haunt me. It reminded me of thousands of mothers in Nigeria who would have no place to turn to get help for their own children. I felt a need to respond.

Millar returned in the afternoon to say, "I am afraid you are going to decide to go back. Could we figure out a way to make this a win for all of us? Why don't you go back for ninety days and develop a program to respond to the needs of refugees in war areas and the CDC could agree to provide a series of people to continue implementing the program?"

Millar was a creative administrator, and the idea was potentially a good solution. In September 1968, Paula and I returned to Nigeria with sons David and Michael for an intense and disturbing three months.

At least Nigeria was familiar. I did not need to start from scratch. We moved into an apartment in Lagos, at that time the capital of Nigeria, registered David in school, and began living in conditions superior to any we had known during our previous times in Nigeria. We not only had electricity and running water but also air-conditioning. We contacted Lawrence Atutu, who had worked with us when we lived in Ogoja Province, to see whether he would help us for three months. He was eager to help but reluctant to fly to Lagos. He finally agreed to, which made it much easier to establish a temporary household in Lagos.

His reluctance to fly had a history. The Ogoja area, where we had previously lived, had no airstrip at that time so planes were only viewed as they occasionally flew over the area. One day a pilot was ferrying a small plane from Lagos to the Republic of Cameroon when he realized his fuel consumption exceeded his expectations. He began searching for a place to land and decided the soccer field in Ogoja town would be adequate. On landing, his wheel hit the top of a yam hill just before the intended touchdown. The plane flipped on its back and skidded down the soccer field on its top. The pilot exited the plane unhurt, but the local children, Lawrence included, thought that was the way planes landed, and he wanted no part of that experience.

Not only were we entering a known environment but also the CDC Smallpox Regional Office was in Lagos, so I could count on help from familiar CDC faces, such as George Lythcott, public health advisor Jim Hicks, and Rafe Henderson. Rafe was fluent in French, well spoken, and persuasive and would later introduce rigorous evaluation techniques into the program. After smallpox, he headed up the WHO global immunization program.

We lived in Lagos, but the actual fieldwork was in Eastern Nigeria. I divided my time between the ICRC headquarters in Lagos and refugee programs at the perimeter of the war area.

Never have I lived amid such chaos. Telephones rarely worked in Lagos, so in-person conversations required driving to another office. Traffic was heavy, making travel such a time-consuming process that essential communications were often lacking. Getting real-time information from the field was difficult, so planners and logistics experts were always working with old information. Military requirements of the Nigerian army received top priority for transportation and communications; local government bureaucrats and military commanders regarded relief work as a burden.

The essential information needed to plan relief operations was unknown. This included such factors as the number of people in each location, their nutritional status, availability of water, amount of food in storage or in transit to each place, a system for decisions on food distribution, number of people in homes versus refugee camps, the presence of infectious diseases such as measles, tuberculosis or meningitis, malaria transmission, and the like. When I saw an order for intravenous protein solutions (an approach already shown to be ineffective and inefficient in times of famine by Ancel Keys during World War II), I realized I needed more knowledge if there was any chance of becoming part of the solution.

In my hurry to get to Nigeria, I only had time to contact some knowledgeable people to ask what information I needed. During World War II, Dr. Keys, at the University of Minnesota, had conducted studies with conscientious objectors to understand the speed of starvation effects but also the best ways of rehabilitation. I collected more information than I could read, hoping to review it on the trip and while in Nigeria. I also collected information on the well-documented famine in the Netherlands during World War II and the incredibly detailed information available on starvation in Leningrad in 1941 and 1942. A major portion of my luggage was eventually occupied by literature on malnutrition, infectious disease outbreaks during famine, and the results of past relief operations. The feeling of being in over my head was becoming familiar. It was the same feeling I had when I started my internship, the EIS program, the smallpox investigation in New Mexico, my stint as Peace Corps physician in India, the immersion into a rural health program in Nigeria, and now a relief operation.

Despite the pressures to make decisions, I deliberately went into seclusion for thirty-six hours and read all of the materials in my suitcase. After that, I felt more confident about what needed to be done but not more confident that it *could* be done.

Surveillance Systems

We began a public health approach to famine and developed forms to be completed by a refugee worker each week at each location. Setting up a surveillance system was daunting. In a relief action, everyone is overstretched and suspicious of extra work or directives coming from elsewhere. Everyone uses surveillance systems all the time to evaluate what they are and should be doing, but they don't think of them as surveillance systems. And they may not realize the importance of a system that cannot only provide information on trends over time but also allow for comparison with other geographic areas. If workers in relief efforts have never worked with public health programs, they may not realize that knowing the truth is the first lesson in appropriate reactions.

The forms were simple because we knew these workers were overworked and would have no patience for requests for any information that they felt was not needed. The forms called for estimates of the number of people in their catchment area, divided by adults and children, in camps or in villages, and the number they were actually feeding. The forms asked for information on the amount of food distributed, children versus adults, the kinds of food, and the amount in storage. Also included was a table of diseases asking for a tally of the number of cases seen that week for adults and children. We included only the diseases for which a response was possible. Of course, we wanted much more information, but if we could not respond we could not ask them to take time to report. It was essential that we know whether smallpox cases were seen (none were during the war because we had stopped the last outbreak in that area the week that fighting started). Information on measles was needed because of the high mortality from that disease in malnourished children. If a response to a reported case of measles would be needed, we could get measles vaccine, jet injectors, and knowledgeable operators. We could also respond to meningitis with antibiotics and isolation, diarrheal disease with oral rehydration therapy, and malaria with chloroquine. The list was short but essential.

I should note that two cases of suspected smallpox were reported from within the enclave of Biafra, but, in both instances, specimens from the patients were flown out on the night flights that provided food. In both cases, the rash was found to be due to vaccinia rather than smallpox. (Both cases were shown to be the result of the strain of vaccine used in the area.)

In this area of Nigeria, measles had routinely killed about 7 percent of all children born, even during peacetime. Mortality rates as high as 25 percent had been reported during the seasonal famine period, that is, during the weeks before first harvest, when food supplies were often scarce. Mortality rates as high as 50 percent had been reported during major famine periods. A vaccine had been tested during the previous decade in Africa; it was so effective that it had been included as the second arm of the Smallpox Eradication Program that the CDC was implementing in West and Central Africa. Because of that program, headquartered in Lagos, we knew we would have no problem in responding quickly. Indeed, when measles was reported in one camp, the response was so rapid that the outbreak was halted within weeks, perhaps the first time a measles outbreak had been aborted as the result of a vaccine response.

Providing food is not a simple task. There is a common belief that if you are hungry enough you will eat anything. The fact is that, in severe starvation, unaccustomed foods will often lead to nausea, vomiting, and diarrhea. However, the preferred food in the area, yams, was so heavy that it was difficult to provide logistically. Grains were donated by many countries and became a staple of the operation. Dried fish from Scandinavian countries was high in protein, easy to incorporate into soups, and similar to pre-famine diets (and therefore well liked). Often countries and organizations would send what was readily available with no knowledge of its acceptability. A shipment of ambrosia (not the food for the Gods depicted in *Homer* but, rather, a tinned fruit salad) was not well tolerated by starving people unaccustomed to the food. It was one of the few donations that could be stored anyplace without a requirement for locks or security. Even hungry people did not steal it.

The surveillance system helped to bring some order to where food would be shipped and helped document how it would be used. But there was no shortage of problems. How would we measure malnutrition with enough precision to use the result to allocate scarce supplies? How would we decide on the use of those supplies? To target certain groups within a geographic area could lead to conflict. To bypass some geographic areas could also lead to conflict.

Height-and-weight tables are helpful in measuring malnutrition in children. Some felt we could only use them if we had height-and-weight tables that were specific for Nigeria. It was soon accepted that they would differ from Western standards only if chronic malnutrition were involved; getting that information might identify the actual nutritional status but would provide no help in meeting the current problem. The relief action could only respond to the current crisis; it could not reverse chronic malnutrition.

Estimates of the malnutrition status of a population could be obtained in several ways. One sign of malnutrition involves swelling of the ankles as serum protein levels decline and the permeability of capillaries increases. Edema surveys by age and sex are useful indicators of the nutritional status of the population in general, under famine conditions. They won't always identify those who are in need of nutritional supplements, however, as edema can be caused by conditions other than malnutrition. Nonetheless, an edema survey is a good tool for estimating the nutritional status of a population in times of severe food shortages.

Another approach is to have the nutritional status of children under about 6 years of age serve as a surrogate for the nutritional status of the population. Cultural factors intervene to some degree. In West Africa, children would often suffer more during the seasonal famine period because adults had to have a certain nutritional level to work the fields and harvest crops if the children were to be fed. The Netherlands, however, spared children as much as possible during the famine that accompanied World War II. The Dutch kept exquisite records of their attempts to respond to the famine. Their results became useful as we struggled to help in Nigeria.

In Eastern Nigeria, the amount of food available during the war years never came close to meeting the needs of the people. A triage system that had some objectivity had to be developed. In refugee camps, all of the people would get food, but at basic minimal levels. Providing shelter, waste disposal, and safe water was also important.

But what could be done for people still living in villages, who had less food than usual and less support of other kinds? It was to everyone's advantage to help them stay in their villages to reduce their risk of illness. Refugee camps often spawn infectious disease outbreaks because of crowding. In villages, it was decided to use children as the indicator of food needs for the family. Children under about 6 years of age were the measurement target.

To understand the nutritional status of children, three measurements are needed—height, weight, and age. Children short for their age are classified as chronically malnourished. Children below weight for their height are acutely malnourished. And children short for their age and underweight for their height have both chronic and acute malnutrition. The problem, of course, is determining the age of most children in African war areas is not possible. However, whatever the past history of malnutrition, children below a certain weight for their height are acutely malnourished, and that is the condition to which relief groups can respond. So the absence of age turned out to be no problem in relief operations.

The measurement techniques were admittedly crude. We would enter a village and set up four stations. At the first station, a child was given a slip of paper and, by means of a carpenter's ruler attached to a wall, the child's height was measured and recorded on the slip. At the second station, the child's weight, as recorded on a bathroom scale, was entered on the paper. At the third station, which used a table that compared heights and weights, children were provided with a food card if their weight fell below a standard for their height. This card permitted food for the child's entire family. At the fourth station, a child received a smallpox vaccination with a jet injector. Jet injectors provided a reliable delivery system, and the child was effectively marked for several weeks or more, as a pustule and then a scab formed, which excluded admission to the line again in that village or a neighboring village, in an attempt to get another food card.

Errors were likely, but the thinking was that if a child was sufficiently nourished, the family had figured out a system for obtaining food. They might even have been diverting it from the relief operations. But whatever the reason, they were not in the dire straits of children falling below that nutritional threshold. A Quaker team later simplified these steps by using arm circumference as a surrogate for weight, thus avoiding the need for scales. They called it the QUAC stick (Quaker arm circumference measuring stick) method.

The CDC Commitment

With a system in place, the next need was to establish continuity in the public health approach to famine. The CDC agreed to replace me with Dr. Lyle Conrad and thereafter with EIS officers. Lyle was the perfect choice since he had worked in Nigeria with the Peace Corps and was the supervisor of the EIS field staff. This connection allowed him to choose officers and share his own experience with them as he briefed them for the assignment. It provided continuity beyond 1968, through 1969, and through the end of the war in January 1970. It was a proud moment for the EIS Program as officers provided assistance under difficult conditions. It was also a sad moment as the EIS lost its first officer in the line of duty, when Dr. Paul Schnitker died in a plane crash on November 20, 1969, as his plane approached Lagos.

The CDC provided two dozen EIS officers over almost two years to maintain the operation. It was the first large-scale international disaster response by the EIS and an experience that led some into pursuing global health careers after their EIS years. Alex Langmuir, at the next EIS conference, rose at the end of my presentation on the program and said he had been opposed to using EIS officers in this way, but he had now become a convert. He now felt it was appropriate and that the introduction of applied epidemiology and surveillance had made a difference in the approach to famine in Nigeria and for future famines.

Most of the CDC people worked in areas that had been retaken by the federal troops. However, during this time, Karl Western, an EIS officer from the class of 1967, volunteered to fly into the enclave. The area of Biafra was slowly being reduced in size. Western was to evaluate the nutritional status in the areas still held by Biafra. His studies showed alarming rates of malnutrition in all age groups. While malnutrition was a serious problem in areas now held by the federal government, the conditions within Biafra were unbelievably serious.

The US State Department was strongly inclined to discount this degree of malnutrition. The thinking seemed to be that, if the problem were as bad as reported, the United States would need to respond; yet, it had sided with Nigeria's federal government. Therefore, the State Department did not want to respond to the nutritional crisis within rebel-held areas.

I was traveling to areas now in the hands of federal troops to evaluate how the relief action was coping. Malnutrition was rampant; many children showed signs of *kwashiorkor*. (This term, from Ghana, describes protein/calorie malnutrition in small children, often resulting in a reddish tint to their hair.) On my return to Lagos from one such trip, I was asked to join embassy members and a visiting State Department official for lunch. The State Department official took me totally by surprise as he informed the embassy staff that much of what was written in the media concerning the plight of civilians in Eastern Nigeria was erroneous. He assumed a false air of authority as he talked about a tribe in Africa that had red hair naturally rather than as the result of malnutrition. He said photographers had taken pictures in that area and then presented them as being taken of children with kwashiorkor in Eastern Nigeria.

I could not have been more astonished by this lack of knowledge and attempt to fabricate. I pulled from my pocket two Polaroid pictures of a boy of perhaps 10 years of age. He had one of the most severe cases of malnutrition I had ever seen in someone still standing. He lacked visible muscle mass and appeared to literally have skin stretched over bones; every detail of his knee and pelvic bones was revealed. His eyes stared out from a skull that had patches of discolored hair. I passed the pictures around and said, "I took these pictures three days ago. Starvation in Eastern Nigeria is real." It hurt

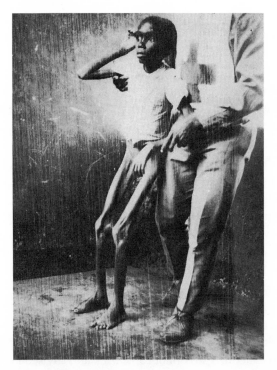

Child in refugee camp, Nigeria, 1968. Photo by the author

to know State Department intelligence could be so driven by ideology rather than the facts.

Years later, I visited the Central Intelligence Agency (CIA) to ascertain what information it might have on smallpox that we were missing. The result was that we discovered we had more information than the CIA did. In the process of discussions, I mentioned my concern about the information the State Department received during the Nigerian Civil War. I told CIA agents that I was happy to have never been debriefed because we always worried about CDC workers being thought of as interested in politics rather than in health. Nevertheless, I said that, to my knowledge, I was the only American in the areas just liberated, and I was curious why no one ever asked for a debriefing. Two of the CIA employees glanced at each other in a way that let me know there was a story. They then told me they had gone to my superior, David Sencer, director of the CDC, for permission to talk to me. He declined, saying that the CDC had to protect its reputation as concerned with health only, not politics or US policy. I was proud of him and proud of the CIA for not pursuing the approach.

The work was gut-wrenching in many ways. Starving people are too weak to revolt. They are lethargic and unable to rouse themselves to effective action. To step over the body of a child who lies where he died is unlike any experience in medicine. I had the constant feeling that I was letting people down.

And there is fear. On one occasion, a small group of Red Cross workers found themselves detained by federal troops. As things appeared to be getting sorted out regarding their authority and where they were working, a soldier suddenly opened fire on them and killed them. This was in my mind as I rounded a corner one day in a Land Rover and a machine gun opened up. There is no good and logical decision in such a case. Stopping and backing up leaves one vulnerable but so does continuing on. We continued on and made it with only our nerves shot.

Another time, I was flying to Enugu as the only passenger in a small plane. We flew over areas of fighting, but the pilot was nonchalant. At one point, he fell asleep. Later, when I pointed out that we were being shot at and tracers were visible, he shrugged it off, saying, "They are terrible shots."

On another occasion, I secured a ride on a DC-6 from Port Harcourt back to Lagos. The plane was returning wounded from the war zone to military hospitals. There were no seats, and the wounded lay on pallets on the floor. I settled in, sitting on the floor with my back against the wall and began reading before takeoff. The copilot came back and advised me to move forward because I was close to the door, and he said it had opened during flights on several occasions.

A young man kept pacing the plane, stepping between the wounded, and he looked agitated. I got up to talk to him and learned that he was a mechanic on contract from Germany. His agitation was caused by the fact that they would not give him time to adequately do repairs. For example, he said, this plane with four engines has only one good generator, and they would not halt long enough for him to repair the other three. He said he had only a few weeks left on his contract, and he was concerned he would not complete the time without an accident. In fact this plane crashed on take-off some weeks later when the only functioning generator failed, killing all on board.

In 1969, Karl Western, Dave Sencer, and I were asked to brief Dr. Henry Kissinger, at that time the national security advisor to President Richard Nixon, on the medical conditions in the Nigerian War area. We were scheduled to see him in the late afternoon, but he fell behind, and we did not actually get a chance to brief him until about 7 p.m. I expected we would be hurried through so he could get back on track, but I was surprised at his deliberate approach in hearing us out as he asked questions.

Kissinger then did something that impressed me beyond belief. He sat down in an easy chair, rubbed his eyes, and said, "For me, those are simply numbers. For you, they must be faces."

The US government became more vocal about starvation in the war areas, and I was sent back to Lagos to brief the ambassador on the Kissinger meeting. I arrived early on a Sunday morning, was picked up at the airport, and was given no opportunity to go to a hotel to wash up. Instead, I was driven directly to the ambassador's residence to brief him that morning. This new interest by the US government was welcomed by those in the relief action, but it actually came too late in the war to have the desired impact on deaths from starvation.

One postscript to this story. I took the Kissinger remark to heart and often told CDC workers to always see faces behind the graphs. Some years later, in 1978, a global health conference was held in Alma Ata in the Soviet Union. It became famous as the place where the slogan "Health for all by the year 2000" was designed; that slogan was used by the WHO for many years. Senator Edward Kennedy had been invited to deliver a major talk at the conference. I was in Washington, DC, for a meeting when the senator's health staffer, Larry Horowitz, called me to tell me about the meeting and to ask whether I would come by his office to review the senator's speech to make comments and suggestions. He said they could not let a copy out of the office. I agreed to stop on my way to the airport.

I reviewed the speech and suggested some additions to consider, and the Kissinger remark came to mind. It is unlikely that a Democratic senator would have quoted Dr. Kissinger, but the thought was so good that I wanted to see it used. So I wrote into the speech, "As a philosopher once said, 'For me, those are simply numbers, but for you in the audience they must be faces.'" They liked it and retained the line.

Some years later, we were having dinner in Atlanta at the home of Gisela and Wolf Bulle. Stuart Kingma, who worked with the World Council of Churches on its health programs, attended. During a summary of his work, Kingma happened to mention attending the Alma Ata meeting and hearing Senator Kennedy speak. He said he couldn't remember much about the speech, but it had been worth attending because of one phrase, "For me, those are simply numbers, but for you in the audience they must be faces." He said Senator Kennedy had nailed it!

Forty years later, much has changed in famine and disaster response, and much remains the same. The changes include attempts to predict famine by monitoring food prices, rain forecasts, and food stocks. Famines today are person made, that is, the result of a political defect such as war, not nature, and because of that, they can largely be predicted, and the world has the capacity to respond. Where response is inadequate, it usually points to a political defect or war.

Bangladesh Cyclone

It has also become standard to evaluate rapidly through quick-and-dirty surveys to understand what is needed before unleashing major responses. Soon after the Nigerian Civil War, a cyclone in Bangladesh almost led to a major US response with field hospitals and X-ray machines. Dave Sencer, at the CDC headquarters in Atlanta, and Henry Mosley and Al Sommer, in Dacca (both former EIS officers), were able to do a fast field survey. They found that, unlike with earthquakes or other disasters, the problems from cyclones were not usually injuries. These researchers did find what Al Sommer termed a *cyclone syndrome*. This consisted of abrasions on the chest and inner arms and thighs due to clinging to trees during the storm. Mosley and Sommer also found that shelter, food, farm implements, and means of rebuilding were lacking after cyclone disasters. The surveyors recommended a response of shelter, hand tools for farmers, seed and fertilizer, and supplies to restock medical facilities to get the society responding quickly. Field hospitals would have had limited usefulness, they noted.

Sencer, Mosley, and Sommer then conducted a more sophisticated survey to better describe the problem and its geographic extent. Their survey was based on years of development at the CDC. Polling is now so common that we often forget the history and the science behind it. People often dismiss political polls, for example, saying, "No one has ever polled me." And yet these polls are able, on the basis of a few thousand interviews, to predict how millions will vote within a relatively small margin of error.

Two statisticians at the CDC, Robert E. Serfling and Ida L. Sherman, had developed ways of taking random samples of people to predict, for example, recent illness, beliefs about immunization, and vaccination levels. When Rafe Henderson was about to conduct a survey of smallpox vaccination rates in Northern Nigeria in the late 1960s, he sought the help of Don Eddins, a statistician working with the Smallpox Eradication Program at the CDC. Eddins had been raised in Texas and had lightning reflexes. He likely could have played major league baseball, but he decided to apply his reflexes to statistics.

Sherman and Serfling based their approach on studying census information, tax records, financial data, and other evidence mined by population statisticians. Eddins transferred their basic approach to areas that lacked street addresses or census numbers and suggested studying people in random clusters rather than identifying random people. A cluster was identified by selecting a random spot on the map. The nearest village was visited, and rules were established on how to choose the first household and the following households in the cluster. Eddins's method became a standard approach in health programs in Africa. Years later when I visited a clinic in Congo Brazzaville and asked how they knew the immunization rates that were posted on the wall, they answered that they used the Henderson method, which was really the Henderson-Eddins method.

Mosley and others now used this approach in the cyclone-hit areas of Bangladesh, with a ferry as base and speedboats to find the clusters. Their survey indicated that 250,000 persons had died in one night because of the cyclone. Deaths were far more frequent than nonfatal injuries. These results reinforced the need for food, shelter, utensils, and farm animals to rebuild the area.

The use of surveillance (including surveys), analysis, and appropriate response has become ingrained in disaster relief. What has not changed is the overwhelming response from countries and nongovernmental organizations (NGOs) that often cause gridlock at airports, often with materials that are of no use for the disaster. Such materials, in fact, become one more burden for relief workers. Human nature dictates competition to get supplies to the area of need and publicizing the work for the benefit of donors. The government, however, not only has an unprecedented disaster to deal with but now politics as well. Such situations often lead to government workers, who should be focused on the disaster, instead attempting to meet the needs of foreign diplomats and representatives of NGOs, who are seeking an audience with those in charge of the disaster.

A lesson that seems difficult to learn is that all resources from outside of the disaster area should be coordinated by one outside person. Often the best person to consider is a military logistician accustomed to moving large volumes of material as efficiently as possible. The government response in the affected country should also be centralized under a single person. These two people—one representing the government, the other representing all outside agencies—could coordinate for maximum effectiveness. Sufficient examples of how to do this exist, as, for example, in the coordination of North Atlantic Treaty Organization (NATO) troops. Yet disasters often catch governments by surprise, and they do not easily respond in an efficient manner. The West African Ebola outbreak is the latest example of the inability of public health and disaster agencies to learn the lessons that seem second nature to military organizations.

chapter 12

SMALLPOX CLAIMS ITS
LAST VICTIMS

When Don Millar took over domestic service programs at the CDC in 1970, including immunization, I took his place as director of the Smallpox Eradication Program. Once again, we were pleased to be back in Atlanta at a crucial time medically. Our third son, Robert, was born at Emory, and on the same day, he was transferred to Egleston Children's Hospital with hyaline membrane disease. He made a full recovery, but we were reminded that such facilities are not available to parents in many parts of the world.

The CDC continued to share its experience and knowledge with other WHO-sponsored programs around the world. The experience of concentrating on the smallpox virus to direct vaccination activities to the most efficient places worked in other geographic areas also. Consistently, focusing on a new area would eliminate the virus. This usually occurred in less than twelve months after a change in strategy to concentrate on surveillance/containment.

Leo Morris, a statistician from the CDC, had been assigned to work in Brazil. Working with Ciro de Quadros, the physician who headed the Brazil smallpox program, they concentrated on surveillance/containment, and soon Brazil became smallpox free. With that event, an entire hemisphere was free of the disease. The CDC also continued to contribute people to the WHO for assignments to countries around the world.

93

Smallpox Vaccine Risks

It was then time to deal with unnecessary deaths due to smallpox vaccine use in the United States. Physicians Mike Lane and John Neff, both former EIS officers, had exhaustively studied the toll of smallpox vaccine in the United States. One person in the United States died about every other month as the result of receiving a smallpox vaccination. In addition, many persons were hospitalized for complications that included a generalized infection from the vaccine, neurologic complications, and, in some cases, the continuing growth of the virus locally, eventually requiring amputation of an arm.

The fear of smallpox in this country was so great that this vaccine carnage had been acceptable in the past. But now it was time to reevaluate and to have the best risk data available, especially if we were to suggest halting infant smallpox vaccination. In 1965, a review at the beginning of the WHO program found forty-three countries endemic with smallpox; that is, smallpox transmission was continuous within the country. This review clarified several issues. Spread of smallpox from those forty-three countries to nonendemic countries induced great fear, but the importations could be stopped. Indeed, it was possible to predict how many generations of smallpox, as well as the number of cases, might follow a new introduction. Second, rough estimates of the risk of exporting smallpox from disease-endemic countries could be calculated on the basis of the incidence of smallpox in each country and the volume of traveler traffic in and out of the country. The higher the incidence of smallpox in a country, the greater the risk for exportation. Also, the greater the volume of traffic from that country, the greater the risk of a traveler's reaching another country with smallpox.

But a third factor also became obvious: Europe appeared to act as a filter for the United States. In those days, there were far fewer direct flights from the United States to Africa or Asia. Europe, therefore, continued to have importations, while the United States had recorded no importations of smallpox since 1949. Travelers from Africa and Asia often stopped for some time in Europe before continuing their travel to the United States. If they were in the incubation period of smallpox, they would likely develop symptoms in Europe before continuing their trip.

The loss of seven people a year in the United States due to the smallpox vaccine increasingly seemed too high a price to pay for smallpox freedom. Theoretically, an importation might lead to ten to twenty cases of smallpox and perhaps six deaths. However, it would require an importation every year to equal the adverse impact then resulting from the domestic smallpox vaccination program. While an importation and even one death would bring critics to the forefront, arguing that we had not protected the public, discussions with the Advisory Committee on Immunization Practices, state health officers, and state epidemiologists finally led to the conclusion that we must take this action, even while smallpox continued to rage, especially in India, Pakistan, and Bangladesh.

Case Manual

With the help of Seth Leibler, head of training at the CDC, an ingenious program was implemented. Training workers in every state would be time consuming and ephemeral. The turnover of staff and the loss of skills not used would require a continuing training program beyond the capacity of the CDC. So Leibler and his staff developed a program called Comprehensive Action in a Smallpox Emergency (CASE).

A large notebook contained a folded diagram that would be unfolded and affixed to a wall in the state or county experiencing a suspected or known case of smallpox. The chart was called a PERT chart (program evaluation and review technique) and used techniques developed by the US Navy in the 1950s to outline the critical path of decisions and actions required to reach an objective. The PERT chart allowed the state or local health department staff to see, step by step, the actions required. It meant that all of the essential steps could be taken at first suspicion of a smallpox emergency, even before the CDC could deploy a person or a team. The training consisted of a visit to every state health department to walk through the steps, put the chart on the wall, and provide familiarity with how the health department staff would respond.

Now, of course, the entire procedure would be online, saving the on-site visits. Yet there was something important in visiting each state, seeing who would be given responsibility, and having them identify with the person they would call on in an emergency.

The full procedure was never implemented. To the credit of the modelers, who could demonstrate that the risk of smallpox was very low in the United States, even while it existed elsewhere, we had no importations. However, the early parts of the PERT chart were used repeatedly while ruling out the possibility of smallpox in a traveler with a rash.

A traveler on a plane arriving with a suspicious rash would be isolated in a holding room at the airport. Specimens of the lesions would be obtained and hand-carried to Atlanta. (The importance of the diagnosis dictated the extra cost of a person's traveling with the specimens to eliminate the chance of specimens being lost.) When the specimen arrived at the CDC, day or night, Jim Nakano, a virologist heading the CDC smallpox laboratory, would personally examine the specimen. Nakano developed the first smallpox lab in the United States and diagnosed the world's last naturally occurring case of smallpox, in a person in Somalia. (There were two laboratory-acquired cases in the United Kingdom following global eradication.) He and his staff would immediately take the specimens, prepare them, and then examine them under an electron microscope. He would attempt to grow viruses from the specimen, but he was so confident of the electron microscope examination that he would provide a preliminary diagnosis within several hours of the specimen's arrival. It was then possible to release the traveler from isolation at an airport. In the meantime, foreign quarantine workers would have identified every person on the flight, with a forwarding address, in the event they had to be vaccinated.

In India

In the summer of 1973, along with Paula and our three sons, David, Michael, and Robert, I went to India, working under the auspices of the WHO.

I benefited from the short-term volunteers Millar freely provided from his workforce to work in smallpox eradication in various countries. (The Bureau of State Services, which he headed, was the largest service-delivery program at the CDC, providing domestic immunizations, tuberculosis and sexually transmitted disease screening, dental work, and other activities, so he had an enormous public health workforce, not only in Atlanta but in all of the states.) Work in the field was a constant problem-solving experience. If an outbreak required more guards placed at the homes of smallpox patients to vaccinate visitors, the CDC short-term volunteer would hire day laborers or borrow people from other health programs. If smallpox patients attempted to leave their home to get food, the CDC person was authorized to provide food services. Rumors of new smallpox cases would trump the plans for that day as the CDC worker figured out how to pursue the rumors.

Workers would return to the United States exhausted but energized with a feeling of accomplishment. Millar once wrote to say he had no idea whether they were helping in the fight against smallpox but to please continue to ask for them. He said that they came back different people, intolerant of roadblocks and focused on solving problems.

India agreed to implement the search-and-containment strategy with the first search involving four states for six days in October 1973. It was a shock, during what was the low transmission season, to find 10,000 new cases of smallpox in two states—cases unknown to the authorities. It overwhelmed our ability to respond with containment. Within six months, India mastered both the search for cases and the response to contain those outbreaks. Soon villages were searched, house by house, and tens of thousands of health workers contained outbreaks. At one time, there were more than 6,000 pending outbreaks, and a single state, the state of Bihar, was discovering 1,500 new smallpox cases a day, one new case each minute.

From a peak of more than 11,000 cases of smallpox reported in a single week in a single state, in May 1974, India went to zero cases of smallpox in the entire country in twelve months.

This may be the most dramatic twelve-month period ever recorded in public health history.

chapter 13

COMING INTO THE UNITED STATES

New Americans

Most people in this country descend from New Americans. The reasons are multiple and complex. Some New Americans came here for adventure, but most came seeking a better life.

In weather systems, low-pressure areas determine where the wind will go next. In a sense, certain areas at certain times in history become low-pressure areas, attracting the winds of change and with them, new immigrants in search of perceived opportunities. The same dynamic operates within a country. In this country, better opportunities pulled people westward, and when the opportunities were perceived to be exceptional, the barometer reading in that area plunged, and people flocked in. The California Gold Rush and the Oklahoma land grants are examples. As the playing field levels, migration patterns subside or even reverse. Once Norwegians flocked to Minnesota and Seattle, for example, but with a level playing field, where skills and knowledge can be applied as easily in one place as in another, people prefer to be with family and familiarity. Someday, that may be the case globally.

But for now, immigration is still robust to the United States. Health officials have attempted over the years to dictate certain conditions that need to be treated in order to allow a person into the country. (Author afternote: When this was written, I could not have even imagined attempts to reduce immigration on the basis of religious beliefs. Civilization is indeed a thin veneer.) At times health officials have even attempted to exclude people with certain conditions. That usually turns out to be counterproductive because people attempt to enter without having the condition detected. Attempts to exclude HIV-positive persons demonstrate this problem.

I write this on April 30, 2013, exactly thirty-eight years after the fall of Saigon. In April 1975, my family returned to Atlanta after working for several years on smallpox eradication in India. I was anticipating a period of decompression, but history intervened. America withdrew from the Vietnam War that April 30 and provided a destination for many who had helped the United States during the war. Dave Sencer asked me to oversee the public health aspects of the refugee influx.

Thousands left Vietnam for an uncertain future. The fear and anxiety that they felt are not possible for us to understand. Some were separated from other family members and so faced the unknown without those who could have given the most support. They were destined for weeks of new locations, uncertainty, health inspections, and often little input into their ultimate destination in the United States.

By May 3, 1975, more than 77,000 refugees had passed through two staging areas, the largest in Guam, the other on Wake Island. CDC assignees were assisting military medical personnel in the health screening at each staging area. The routine became for them to call Atlanta each day to report on the number of refugees in residence, the number arriving in the previous twenty-four hours, the number departing to the US mainland, and the health status of those screened. As with the Nigeria/Biafra relief program, a surveillance system was developed to characterize the size of the health problems and to provide assistance in resolving those problems.

About 30,000 of the 77,000 had already arrived in the United States at one of three military bases—Camp Pendleton in California, Fort Chaffee in Arkansas, and Eglin Air Force Base in Florida. About 9,000 of the 30,000 had been discharged to relatives or sponsors and had left for their final destinations.

Health problems were less significant than many had feared. About 3 percent of persons arriving at the staging areas were hospitalized, most for pneumonia, gastroenteritis, or obstetric reasons. In the first 77,000 screened, no diseases required quarantine, and only two cases of malaria, one case of typhoid fever, and a dozen cases of tuberculosis were found. Because of cases of measles, an active immunization program was initiated in the staging areas and in the US military camps.

When a destination was established for a refugee family, the state health department was provided with the chest X-rays, serologic results for syphilis, immunization records, and a record of health problems detected, especially those that required follow-up. An attempt was made to minimize time in camps to avoid communicable diseases and to facilitate refugees in obtaining the stability of a final location. For some refugees, departure to their final destination could be accomplished in days once they reached mainland camps. For many, their time in camps would be measured in weeks, but others remained for months before they reached a final destination. If the health screenings on the US military bases would cause undue delay, the Immigration and Naturalization Service arranged for the exams to be conducted at the refugees' final destination.

The *MMWR*, the CDC's weekly newsletter, provided frequent summaries of the findings during the health screenings. It also provided information on recommended treatment, for example, of malaria if it should be detected after a refugee's arrival in a state.

By May 14, more than 111,000 persons had reached the staging areas. Of this number, 56,000 had already arrived on the mainland; 16,000 of these had been released to sponsors. Health problems remained small: 20 cases of malaria and 215 cases of suspected tuberculosis. In retrospect, the flow of individuals was quite efficient.

To speed up processing, a fourth mainland camp was opened on May 28 at Indian Town Gap, Pennsylvania. The entire screening operation had overcome the early problems and was now running with smooth efficiency. The first cases of tuberculosis or leprosy, for example, required a review of how best to handle care and follow-up. Each subsequent case would benefit from the procedures developed. By the end of August, 130,000 persons had arrived, and 75,000 had already been placed with sponsors. Disease counts, although relatively low, continued to increase; 39 cases of Hansen's disease (leprosy) had been diagnosed by the end of the year, and 2,000 persons were diagnosed with possible tuberculosis. But the real news continued to be a relatively healthy population that had entered the country, the efficiency of the operation in general, the openness of the US population in providing sponsorship, and the gratitude expressed by the refugee population. (In 2011, I met a doctor in military uniform who informed me she had been one of those child refugees, and she was now trying to pay her debt to this country.)

Jimmy Carter Becomes President . . . and There Are Consequences

In November 1976, Jimmy Carter became president and selected Joseph Califano, a lawyer who had been an aide to President Lyndon Johnson, as the secretary of the Department of Health, Education and Welfare. One of Califano's first actions as secretary was to ask Dave Sencer to come to Washington, DC. Califano was not happy with the Swine Flu Vaccination Program and put the blame at Sencer's doorstep. My own feelings were that Sencer had acted in the best interest of public health, but that the public health community had been fooled by a virus: for the first time in history, a new strain of influenza that had been shown to be capable of spreading from person to person in a population devoid of antibodies to the strain had *not* resulted in a pandemic.

In any case, Hale Champion, Califano's deputy, informed Sencer that he would have to leave the position. A petition signed by hundreds at the CDC, including me, asked for the department to reconsider, but it did not.

I did not know it at the time, but Dave Sencer had requested that the department include my name in the list of candidates to replace him. My interests were so focused on global health that I had never even contemplated the position of the CDC director until I was asked to submit my

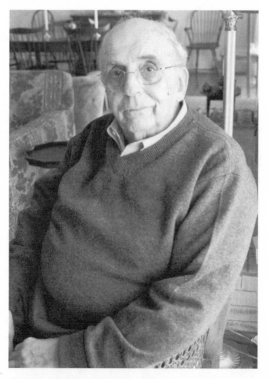

Dr. David Sencer, director of the Centers for Disease Control and Prevention from 1966 to 1977, in 2008. Courtesy of Emory Photo/Video

résumé. I was not eager to do that as I saw it as a diversion from my real interests in global health. Dave asked me to at least go for the interview as a favor to him, pointing out the potential for promoting global health in that position and reminding me of what he had been able to do in that position for smallpox eradication.

I went to Washington for the interview. My ambivalence prevented me from being nervous. For example, when I entered Secretary Califano's office, he was emptying an ashtray, and he apologized. He said that the last guest in his office was a smoker, and he was sorry for the smell. I replied that I was surprised because I had assumed that the secretary had sufficient authority to designate his own office as a smoke-free zone. He

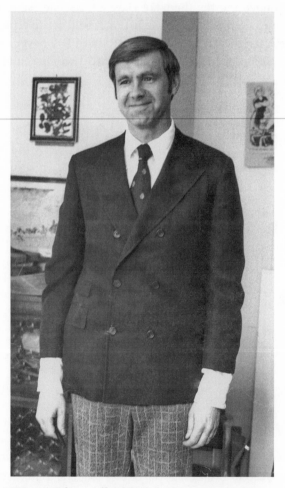

The author in 1976, posing for an official CDC photo. Photo from the CDC

looked startled, and when I returned for a second interview, there was a No Smoking sign in his office.

He called me some time later to say he would like me to be the director of the CDC and that he would personally come to the CDC on Friday to talk to the staff and announce his decision. In the meantime, I was to tell no one but my wife.

Minutes later, even before I had time to call my wife, Don Berreth, director of the Information Office at the CDC, entered my office to say that the information office in HEW had called him, requesting that he prepare a résumé on me and get a photograph. Don told me that he did not want to share this information with anyone else at the CDC and therefore he would take the photo in his office.

I reached for my suit coat, but he said that everyone knew I wore my coat only for guests or special occasions, so to carry the coat to his office might alert someone. So we went to his office, and I put on *his* suit coat. It was far too short, with six inches of shirt showing at the end of the sleeves. Don said it was no problem since he was only getting a head shot.

After taking the picture, Don suggested that, since it was a special occasion, I should get a standing shot to show how ridiculous the jacket looked. He said that he and I would be the only ones to ever see it. I agreed and can only marvel at my naïveté.

On Friday, Secretary Califano came to the CDC and made the announcement. By the end of the day, everyone seemed to have a copy of me standing with Don's suit coat on. His explanation was that of course he meant it when he said that he would not share the picture. But the moment Califano announced my appointment I had become a public figure, and I had lost my privacy. After all, this was the official picture. It was a wonderful joke at my expense and might as well be shared.

chapter 14

ORGANIZING FOR SUCCESS

I had already been associated with the CDC for fifteen years when I was appointed its director. Before, I had always focused on specific problems. Now, I had to think of the entire organization, to ask what we were doing and what we *should* be doing. What did good stewardship come down to on a daily basis?

The National Institutes of Health (NIH) was seen as the research arm of the Public Health Service. The CDC was seen as the delivery arm of public health. Early on, I fortunately met with Don Fredrickson, director of NIH, to discuss how best to position the two agencies when we testified before Congress. I told him that I respected the traditional differences but had also noticed that the most productive employees at the CDC were not only focused on delivery but also always asking how to improve on what they were doing. Therefore, they were involved in research, looking for better tools and better ways of using those tools, and expanding what was known. Dr. Fredrickson said the same was true at NIH: the best researchers were involved in seeing their innovations and discoveries used. Therefore, they were involved in delivery to improve on the research findings and to guide future research. We concluded that there should be no sharp line between the two agencies and that, within the overall understanding that the CDC was in delivery and NIH in research, we would encourage employees in both organizations to combine research and delivery.

Purpose

Implementing the tools and resources to improve the public's health is easy to understand. However, a daily concern revolved around doing the right things and doing them right. What *were* the right things? Originally, we were charged with targeting infectious diseases, but the mandate was slowly expanding. Our objectives were threefold: we were charged with (1) eliminating premature death, (2) eliminating unnecessary suffering, and (3) improving the quality of life. Eliminating death is not achievable, but defining premature deaths and preventing them can be achieved. The definition continues to change as tools improve, so the CDC's objective was always evolving. Eliminating suffering is also not achievable, but defining what is not acceptable, what is unnecessary suffering, is crucial. Finally, beyond death and physical suffering, there are the problems inherent with poverty, gender bias, illiteracy, unemployment, mental illness, and other social determinants that reduce the quality of life. Public health seeks to alleviate those problems. The tools for achieving these goals with infectious diseases are applicable to many conditions, so it is no surprise that the purview of the CDC continued to enlarge.

Evolution is a word fraught with emotion for many. Because the original task of the CDC was focused on communicable diseases, the staff included many microbiologists, and microbiologists have a front row seat to observe evolution. Viruses and bacteria are continuously changing to adapt to a new environment. Antibiotics were very useful when first introduced. However, bacteria develop countermeasures, often through mutations, to survive in the presence of an antibiotic. Soon those strains predominate, and the antibiotic or antimalarial drug became less useful and, in some cases, totally useless.

But one need not be a microbiologist to understand evolution. When my grandson asked me, "What is the best argument for evolution?" I answered, "The Westminster Dog Show." It is obvious at a glance that dogs have a spectrum of sizes, shapes, looks, and abilities; yet, they have all developed from the DNA of wolves. To make it even more interesting, apparently the wolf group that evolved into modern dogs is extinct. It could not continue to survive as it was.

Many of my teachers emphasized that we are a mixture of nature and nurture. They always maintained that the environment in which we grew molded our basic genetic material, but that environment could not alter the DNA itself. But now, in the twenty-first century, we are learning that the environment can indeed alter DNA, inserting another ingredient into evolution.

Public health itself evolves, and soon it became necessary for the CDC to enlarge the area of concern from only communicable diseases to chronic diseases, such as cancer, heart disease, strokes, and diabetes. Rei Ravenholt (see chapter 5) had argued over the years that death certificates list the obvious clinical causes of death but that they should also list generic causes of the clinical condition, such as tobacco, alcohol, or diet.

Public health advocates kept enlarging their areas of interest. Violence was increasingly seen as a public health problem together with environmental toxins and workplace exposures. Over time, most health problems were found to have public health components. Dr. Yemi Ademola, my classmate from Nigeria in Tom Weller's class at Harvard, used to say, "There is no field of knowledge beyond the interest and concern of public health practitioners."

In 1993, J. Michael McGinnis and I published a paper in the *Journal of the American Medical Association* (*JAMA*) on the actual causes of death in the United States (1). Our conclusion was that, instead of listing heart disease, cancer, and stroke, the actual causes were tobacco (400,000 deaths a year), diet and activity patterns (300,000 deaths), and alcohol (100,000 deaths). These three factors accounted for 40 percent of the deaths in this country.

Yet even that approach is inadequate in explaining death patterns in this country. We need a new article on the causes behind the causes, in an attempt to determine the proportion of deaths due to poverty, lack of education, gender bias, unemployment, and other social determinants of health. The WHO and the CDC have both published on the social determinants of health and deaths, and in 2014, the faculty at Emory University added to the list by editing and publishing a book on religion as a social determinant of health (2).

Structure

Structure follows function, and during the early years of the CDC, with its focus on communicable diseases, the structure followed skill sets. Laboratory programs used bench scientists, who were working on understanding organisms, researching better ways of detecting them, following patterns of resistance to antibiotics, discovering the causes of outbreaks, and finding and characterizing pathogens never before seen.

Epidemiology was another major focus and enlarged greatly with the recruitment of Alexander Langmuir. Statistical programs expanded to support the epidemiologic and laboratory work. At that time, the CDC was small enough that much of the structure was informal and did not require a "structural adjustment." A management expert studying the CDC in the 1960s defined it as a mom-and-pop operation that seemed to work fine.

The problems arose with new outbreaks to be investigated. Each outbreak required a matrix management ad hoc approach, which depended on early guesses as to the organism involved. The problems were always worked out, but there was a cost in efficiency.

As the complexity of public health increased, the CDC was forced to define the high-priority areas of concern. The agency needed to determine what function it should play and how it should be structured to fulfill that function.

I did not face these questions alone. The CDC had a staff of thousands, but beyond that, we all bring with us the input of thousands of others, for we are all truly connected and in the struggle together. John Donne was correct when he wrote (3):

No man is an island,
Entire of its self,
Every man is a piece of the continent,
A part of the main.

The implications go beyond the idea of human connections. A million ancestors have influenced my DNA, just since the Renaissance. Even more have influenced my social DNA.

Social DNA includes the influence of many, directly and, even more, indirectly. Some of the most obvious are those we regard as mentors, people who have had an influence on our thoughts, beliefs, way of working, and sense of responsibility. The list of mentors seems endless. (For my partial list, see the appendix.)

Advice from the Past

Every new position, as medical student, intern, EIS officer, medical missionary, smallpox worker, refugee health coordinator, and now the CDC director, initially made me anxious. Was I prepared? Could I find the right people to provide guidance? How would we choose priorities, develop strategies, and measure our performance? Would we have the courage to acknowledge mistakes, and would we learn from those mistakes?

The wisdom of historical people is invaluable not only because their ideas were often the end product of everything they had learned but also because those ideas could be evaluated in the context of what happened after these people have lived, a perspective obviously denied to them. And so I went back, before going forward. It was similar to the thirty-six hours taken during the Nigerian famine relief operation to absorb the wisdom of the past before being certain about my next steps.

What continued to surprise me was the consistency of the conclusions of great people regarding what constitutes the best ways to live and the consistency of our resistance to adopting their recommendations. They repeatedly praised knowledge and science, while, at the same time, warning of the limitations of science. They consistently promoted social justice, while the world continued to promote slavery and bias. It is easy to get discouraged when faced with the economic inequities in the world, despite the pleas of Amos the prophet. And so I reviewed notes made over the years that provided advice on public health before the discipline even existed.

Polybius was a reminder to me that the world is an organic whole, with everything affecting everything, and that the voices of 100 billion people who have preceded us were still speaking to those who would listen.

Confucius reminded me to emphasize morality and the Golden Rule as a basis for the CDC's responsibility to improve life for all and to be cautious about the power inherent in teaching others how to be healthy. The itch to teach is a part of the itch to rule; scratch the one and find the other. There is a strong need for a social conscience in this organization called the CDC. Imhotep, apparently the first scientist that we know by name, a physician and the builder of the Step Pyramid, would urge us to combine art and science in every endeavor and in every scientist.

The echo of Euripides's songs attacking slavery, gender bias, and aristocracy was a reminder of the need for social equity and urged me to use the CDC's facilities for the poorest people in the poorest countries. Through 2,500 years of history, I could imagine him preaching about the social determinants of health.

That mission was enforced by Arnold of Villanova, physician to James II. I read of his diplomatic missions, where he was shocked by the health, misery, and exploitation of the poor. He did not mince words. He condemned the wealth of the clergy, and, despite being pursued during the

Inquisition, he repeatedly warned the king that unless he protected the poor from the rich he would go to hell.

At a time of increasing specialization, I remembered Averroes, the great Islamic philosopher, lawyer, and physician, who saved for us the works of Aristotle. He was the first to recognize that an attack of smallpox confers immunity and argued for the integration of knowledge from medicine, philosophy, physics, psychology, law, theology, and astronomy.

Roger Bacon would say that he saw the CDC coming 700 years ago. He seems to have seen everything else—cars, airplanes, submarines, and telescopes. But his warning is still clear 700 years later. Science has no moral compass, so scientists must cultivate one.

Rabelais would repeat the ten words that he has Gargantua saying to his son, "Science without conscience is but the ruin of the soul." This should be on the wall of every science department.

Francis Bacon would utter his legendary words, "Knowledge itself is power." But despite his zest for knowledge, Bacon subordinates it to morality. "Of all virtues and dignities of the mind, goodness is the greatest," he wrote.

Benjamin Franklin would be absolutely delighted by the science from the CDC. He once said, "O that moral science was in as fair a way of improvement . . . and that human beings would at length learn what they now improperly call humanity." Franklin lost his son to smallpox, and he would have had a special interest in the CDC.

Albert Schweitzer would remind us that ethics goes beyond people to include animals, plants, and the environment. He would caution all those with any power to be mindful of the destiny that they are creating for others. This remains vital for everyone who will ever work in the CDC's buildings.

Einstein, standing before the Caltech student body (4), said, "It is not enough that you should understand . . . science . . . Concern for the man himself and his fate must always form the chief interest of all technical endeavors . . . in order that the creations of our mind shall be a blessing and not a curse to mankind." But the quote from Einstein that I have used the most over the years is, "Nationalism is an infantile disease. It is the measles of mankind."

The physicist Richard Feynman famously said that time moves in only one direction—that, for example, it takes very little energy to scramble an egg, but all of science is incapable of reversing that simple process. This underscores the importance of the CDC's mission to use science for prevention.

The drumbeat of history could not be ignored: the wisest people of the past agree on the need for social justice, and that means global social justice.

There was no end of advice from the past, but it was also important to get advice from the present. So, with these lessons from unmet mentors firmly ingrained, we sent out a letter to national, state, and local health officers, as well as to academic institutions and many others, asking for their input on what they regarded as the most important tasks that the CDC should pursue. More than 400 people returned thoughtful responses. Seth Leibler took responsibility for organizing the responses into eighteen different categories. The traditional areas of public health, infectious diseases, sanitation, water safety, health education, and immunization were frequent subjects of the letters. But an expansion of interests was becoming evident. Violence, substance abuse, chronic diseases, genetics, mental health, and disaster relief were also well represented.

We then formed a committee—the Red Book Committee—based on the color of its final report. We asked the members to look at the responses and, on the basis of what was known about suffering and death in this country, to tell us what they thought the CDC's highest priorities should be. All committee members were from outside the agency because the group was advising the CDC, and we did not want insiders influencing the direction their recommendations would take. The one exception was Don Millar, who acted as secretary for two reasons: first, to be the interface with the CDC for any questions the committee might have and, second, to be responsible for the report's acceptance and use at the CDC.

One interesting development was the Red Book Committee's concern that mortality statistics are difficult to interpret because infants and children who die young have equal power in analysis to 90-year-olds who die; thus, children's deaths may not highlight the potential for prevention activities—as they should. From the committee's inquiry came a new approach, still used today, namely, that of premature deaths. How many years are lost before a given age because of early death? It might seem logical to use the median age of death as the cutoff for premature death. The problem is that it would change each year, so it was decided to select an age and continue to use that. What age should be chosen? There were good arguments for selecting age 70 or even 75, but in the end, 65 was selected because global statistics often use that as a standard, and the committee wanted to be able to compare the United States to other countries.

After much discussion, the committee prepared a report on the priority areas it felt should especially concern the CDC.

The CDC followed the publication of the report with two retreats at Berry College in North Georgia, an off-site location close to Atlanta. The retreats were designed to give top management an opportunity to speak for or against the priorities. In the end, the CDC's top managers accepted them all and added a few more. It was agreed that budget requests to the Public Health Service would reflect an annual review of priority areas. The important result was a priority list that had support from all.

Reorganization

Agreeing on how the CDC should be structured was much more difficult. The basic result was an agreement that the CDC should reorganize from an expertise orientation to a health-outcome orientation. For example, we should have a Center for Infectious Diseases that would contain all the expertise needed in laboratory sciences, epidemiology, statistics, social sciences, and other areas for the center director to be able to achieve infectious disease goals. There would be a center for environmental health, one for occupational health, and eventually one for chronic diseases and injury control. Matrix management would still be required for problems that were unclear at the beginning of an investigation, but the new structure made the CDC much more efficient.

With an agreement on a new structure, a new problem arose. Scientists working in the laboratory were concerned that they would not have the same supervision if a bench scientist did not supervise them. One can read that as a lack of confidence in epidemiologists to understand the lab scientists' needs. A large portion of the laboratory force would be in the new Center for Infectious Diseases. Bench scientists had been supervised for so long by people with the same background that they could not easily accept supervision by others. Soon I learned that a number of top scientists were seeking employment in other places, including academic institutions or state laboratories.

It was crucial to have a center director of the Center for Infectious Diseases who could bring a new group of people together in a functioning unit. By the time the first director stepped down, it was hoped that employees of the Center for Infectious Diseases would have worked so effectively that the tension between bench scientists and epidemiologists would have eased. Dr. Walter Dowdle was a virologist, highly respected in the lab but also by epidemiologists. He had a special interest in influenza, and because this was an annual problem, he had worked closely with epidemiologists to determine which strains of virus should be incorporated into the influenza vaccine each year.

I talked to Walt about the position, but he was not interested because he enjoyed bench science. I had always avoided talking people into positions; I thought it important for people to follow their passion, not someone else's desire. Despite that basic belief, I went back to Walt and tried again. I failed. On the third try, he agreed to give it a try, and it solved all of the problems that were brewing. Bench scientists stayed, and Walt had the ability to make a new center work. Best of all, he came to enjoy it. After he retired from the CDC, he continued to work on polio eradication and was successful in developing a global laboratory network capable of isolating, defining, and following polio lines of infection as the world organized to eliminate polio from the globe.

The CDC continued to be a place of wonder. Combining good science with a strong drive for social justice attracted an unusual group. I once remarked that, walking down the hall, it sometimes appeared that we had hired the campus radicals of the 1960s. We had activists who often could not believe that they were working for the government they had recently condemned. But as noted elsewhere, whatever your feelings about government, it is the only institution that represents all of us. No church, social organization, or service club can do that. Therefore, government is the only place that can provide actual social justice for all. It is a revelation for social activists when they finally discover that.

The Workforce

The workforce also evolved and became a combination of several cohorts. There were the scientists, often working in the laboratory, striving to find better ways to study organisms or to detect chemicals in the environment. The scientists tended to be academic in their perspectives, and while some would move on to academic settings, some remained at the CDC for their entire careers. Notable examples included the late Charles Shepard, who focused his disciplined mind on less-studied organisms, such as the bacterium responsible for leprosy. Joe McDade focused on rickettsia and was the scientist to discover the organism that caused Legionnaires' disease. Joe was a leader in forming the online scientific journal *Emerging Infectious Diseases*. In recent years Olen Kew, a gifted virologist, has brought cutting-edge science to the understanding of polioviruses. I believe he actually understands how the poliovirus *thinks*. Walter Dowdle became a legendary figure, as noted. He worked in the laboratory on influenza viruses and became an encyclopedia of knowledge as this virus changed its appearance in a constant attempt to remain relevant and to avoid the threat of whatever influenza vaccine was currently deployed.

A second grouping involved managers. Scientific knowledge is weak in its original state. It must be used to be powerful. As the management consultant Peter Drucker once observed, that means it has to degenerate into work. Management is the work tool that allows knowledge to change the outcomes in public health. Many of the original managers came from the Malaria Control Program of World War II. These were gradually replaced by managers who learned their trade as field-workers in the field of sexually transmitted diseases. This group combined blood-drawing skills with interpersonal skills, honed while interviewing individuals about their sexual activities, and detective skills, refined in finding contacts of persons with a sexually transmitted disease. Their work helped them to develop skills as diplomats and salespeople. Imagine getting a person to share the name of a sexual contact with the reassurance that the information would not become public. These workers had to convince people that they could be trusted.

The venereal disease workers became unusually adept as problem solvers, and they moved on to become accomplished managers of many programs at the CDC. Their ability to keep secrets was profound. Following the death of a famous person with AIDS, identified by news reports as being gay, I chanced to be at a meeting with a dozen of these workers. After the public disclosure, they were free to talk, and it was soon apparent that half of the people in this meeting knew the true situation, had contacted this person regarding other sexually transmitted diseases, and had never shared this knowledge, even with their fellow workers. It was from this background that the late Bill Watson emerged to become deputy director of the CDC and a leader of such integrity that he had the respect not only of the managerial cohort but also of all others in the organization.

There were several other cohorts in the mixture. One consisted of EIS officers, who were recruited for two-year terms as one of the draft options in the CDC's early days. Therefore, at the beginning of EIS, they were all men. Many spent their two years at CDC headquarters; others were assigned to states, cities, counties, or academic institutions. Many stayed beyond their two years, some for entire careers. The CDC had to become even more professional, hiring cutting-edge experts in scientific, training, and managerial fields to support these officers as they investigated outbreaks. The officers, in turn, kept a continuing stream of new ideas coming into the CDC.

Finally, the CDC had an enormous support staff; secretarial support, janitorial services, glass washing, engineering, and computer expertise were among the services provided by over 160 different occupational groups. While the scientists, managers, and EIS officers tended to be recruited from national labor pools, the support staff tended to be recruited from the Atlanta area.

Equal Employment Opportunities

Atlanta in the 1950s and 1960s, as in the rest of the country, was working through the great social changes of the civil rights era. Atlanta had a stability not found in some cities because of its fair-minded and inspirational leaders in the African American community, such as Martin Luther King Jr., Andrew Young, Benjamin Mays, and John Lewis. In the white community, people such as business and civic leader Ivan Allen Jr. led Atlanta through turbulent times when segregationist Lester Maddox was in his political prime. Ralph McGill, editor of the *Atlanta Constitution*, was a strong influence; he featured continuing editorials and articles on the importance of rights, fairness, and diversity not only in Atlanta but also in the rest of the country.

The CDC did not escape the tensions of those years. At one point, an underground newspaper, the *Plantation News*, was published, which complained about the bias inherent in the CDC's hiring practices. Dave Sencer, director of the CDC at the time, wanted no discrimination and sought an approach to equal employment opportunity that was both fair and transparent. A large percentage of the total workforce came from the local community and the CDC needed to make it a representative workforce. Sencer asked me to head up a committee to advise him on the most effective way of making sure that our intentions of equal opportunity were matched by actions.

In those days, the Public Health Service was recommending weekend sensitivity sessions that included employees and their managers. The idea was that everyone could discuss their feelings, complaints, and concerns openly, with no adverse implications when they returned to work on Monday. Sensitivity sessions relied on compartmentalizing thoughts and emotions—workable in theory but difficult in fact.

I went to the American Management Association and asked what experiences their members had in implementing equal employment opportunities and whether they could draw conclusions from those experiences. The association had a database of companies that had tried a spectrum of activities. The most successful approaches had relied on managerial approaches rather than on sensitivity approaches. If achieving a diverse workforce was part of the expectations for managers and was reflected in the evaluation performed by supervisors, and if performance ratings and promotions took that into account, success was more likely. In later years, I realized this was the basis for an observation that "it is easier to change a mind than a heart."

Over forty-two years later, I have gone back to our committee report. It recommended that Dr. Sencer should approach equal opportunity in hiring as a problem to be solved by an organization of problem solvers. Three training sessions were recommended. The first was a series of meetings, starting with Dr. Sencer and all staff reporting to him, and continuing through programs, branches, sections, units, and subunits. The purpose was to establish the philosophy that the CDC was going to solve this problem but that the solutions would come from the programs and move up. The second series of meetings went in reverse, from subunits to the center level, listing the commitments made by each program. Dr. Sencer would not set the goals for the CDC until he had heard from the programs. The purpose was for each manager to make a commitment on the basis of the program's present profile and how the manager thought it could change in three, six, nine, and twelve months. Each manager's plan and commitment would be presented and merged with other commitments as the meetings progressed back to the director's level.

Our assumption, which turned out to be correct, was that the composite plan, reflecting the decisions of managers, would provide targets even higher than if Dr. Sencer started with center-wide targets.

A third series of meetings from subunits to the center level allowed each area to review its commitments now that a plan for the entire CDC existed. This series of meetings also offered a chance for comments to be directed to the center director. These meetings also detailed plans for evaluation, determining what would be measured, how often, and how the results would be distributed. When the third round was complete, the commitment made by each program became clear. Quarterly evaluations would be based on numbers of employees by sex and race at each salary level and within each occupational category, changes in number over time, shortcomings in commitments, and a summary of new hires in each category.

This plan seems so logical at this point in history but, interestingly, the Public Health Service was wary of the approach. However, because of that community's respect for Dr. Sencer, they gave a provisional six-month approval, with a promise to review the results at that time.

At six months, the review, by the office of the assistant secretary for health in the Public Health Service (HEW), was favorable, and the approval was extended. The CDC continued to make good progress in providing opportunities for women and minorities.

Some years later, after I had become director of the CDC, an administrator from the Public Health Service requested a time to talk to the senior staff. He presented a plan for equal employment opportunities for the CDC to implement along with the rest of the Public Health Service. As he was discussing the plan, I realized it was the CDC plan from some years earlier that had been given provisional approval, six months at a time. I sent a note to Carol Walters, who was attending the meeting, asking whether she could go to the files and get a copy of our original plan, which she did. When the Public Health Service administrator finished, I told him he could count on us and then showed him a copy of our original plan, the provisional approval by the Public Health Service, and a summary of how it had worked out. Satisfaction is the word that came to mind.

Daily Operations

Epidemiology can be reduced to the concept of acquiring numerators and denominators to determine a rate and then interpreting that rate. Similarly, public health can be reduced to surveillance systems to acquire information on the health of the public and the use of that information to make decisions that enhance the health of all. Every daily activity in some way supports that core. The surveillance system is then used to determine the impact of the activities to make midcourse corrections. The process continues to be repeated.

Some outbreak accounts have already been related. But what happened at the CDC on a daily basis? Much of the activity involved developing and maintaining usable national and global surveillance systems. This resulted in a continuing flow of information on every health condition imaginable. Originally, the information systems were geared to infectious diseases. Over time, similar systems developed for the entire expanding range of public health. Beyond the conditions reported by all, certain states had special interests in other diseases, and as state epidemiologists make the decisions regarding what they report, there are parallel reporting systems. In addition, state laboratories and many medical laboratories report directly on organisms they have isolated. Current and former EIS officers around the country and around the world are in daily contact. Then and now, there is a whirlwind of activity in the labs and offices as people work on analyzing data, developing new tests, testing the thousands of samples coming to the CDC, and reporting back information to all who need to know. The parallel in clinical medicine involves taking the history of a patient and conducting physical and laboratory examinations. In public health, the surveillance system is continuously taking the history of a community, state, nation, or the world.

In 1950, the first national surveillance system for a single disease, malaria, was established. International treaties had identified a small number of diseases—including smallpox, cholera, plague, and yellow fever—as reportable. The states were expected to report those diseases, but it was largely a passive system. In 1950, the first active surveillance system was established for malaria. It was a surprise when reported malaria cases were tested to find that malaria had quietly disappeared from this country. The second surveillance system was developed in 1955 because the polio vaccine from Cutter Laboratories was causing disease. The surveillance system quickly identified the problem and was able to exonerate vaccines from other manufacturers. The third system was developed in 1957 for influenza. Thereafter, surveillance systems mushroomed, and the CDC always had a point person responsible for each reportable disease.

While public health workers continue to identify the systems as surveillance systems, the word often conjures up the thought of CIA activities. In reality, the programs are attempts to develop disease *intelligence* systems, but surveillance has become the operative word.

The systems, over time, went from infectious diseases to everything imaginable in the area of human health and welfare. Systems now exist for all of the chronic conditions, including heart disease, stroke, and diabetes, but surveillance systems also now exist for tracking factors leading to those problems. Surveillance of weight, blood pressure, smoking rates, and other predictors of health problems is common. Disease problems resulting from occupational or environmental exposures are tracked as well as the chemicals and toxic substances thought to be involved. The data bank has become increasingly sophisticated.

A parallel is seen globally. Famine used to be detected after it was obvious that children were starving. Now surveillance systems exist for rainfall, crop cover, and market prices, providing information on what might happen long before malnutrition is detected. The system for famine detection is now so robust that starvation can be attributed to conflict or political problems rather than to lack of information on the nutritional status of the population.

Collecting the data is only a start. Data must be analyzed to understand the meaning of the information. Analyses are ongoing at different levels and at different speeds. For example, a report of a suspected case of smallpox, cholera, or anthrax leads to immediate analysis and action. Smoking rates, on the other hand, are tracked over time.

Response

Public health is characterized by action. Analysis must lead to some response, either immediate or in the future. While this is widely accepted today, the development of surveillance evolved from archiving, which is simply recording events, to an academic approach, where the events might be analyzed and reported but with no response. Modern public health surveillance uses the entire cycle of collection, analysis, response, and then restarting the cycle with the new information collected.

William Farr was a pioneer in the development of surveillance systems. In the early 1830s, he qualified as a doctor in London and while in practice he became interested in medical statistics. He began working in the General Register Office for England and Wales and developed a system for recording causes of death. This allowed comparisons according to the deceased's occupation, age, and geography.

In 1849, a cholera outbreak in London took the lives of 15,000 people. By examining data from that outbreak, Farr developed theories on how cholera spread. This is the same outbreak that was studied by John Snow, who concluded that the disease was spread by contaminated water. Snow was correct, but Farr thought the disease was spread by air (i.e., the miasmic theory), and he showed over the years that death rates decreased with elevation above the river. For him, this was proof of the theory of air as the vehicle. Although Farr did not accept Snow's theory, Farr helped Snow by providing the addresses of the people who had died, allowing Snow to develop spot maps of the deceased. Years later, Farr's doubts were overcome by good data, and he concluded that Snow was correct in his interpretation, showing once again that doubt and uncertainty provide the basis for sound scientific conclusions.

Now surveillance systems are much more intensive. Many reports are automatically generated as organisms are identified. Google has raised the possibility of estimating influenza activity even earlier than the CDC by analyzing the requests for information on influenza symptoms and the geographic location of those inquiries. However, the "noise" of the Google approach does not make the information more reliable. Real-time analysis of laboratory results, with instant reporting as part of the diagnostic process, will reduce delays and will speed up the analysis. It is possible to foresee a day when urine and stool analysis in public toilets, as well as air analysis in buildings and real-time reporting of individual patient isolations, will provide part of the evaluation of the health of people in the aggregate.

Having reached preliminary judgments about disease patterns, the CDC shares the information in a variety of ways. Informally, report providers are in a constant dialogue.

The Importance of Partnerships

The CDC routine has always involved a weekly publication, the *MMWR*. This provides raw data on a wide variety of diseases, commentary and explanations, and summaries of the science for various conditions. Raw data allow readers to do their own analyses and to keep the system transparent.

At one point, as part of reducing government spending, the administration declared that the CDC must stop sending out the *MMWR* for free. I was concerned about the government's inability to understand that this newsletter was an important part of public health administration, an efferent arm to the surveillance cycle. It is an essential part of transparency to provide information back to those who have provided it, to those who can improve health by having that information, and, in a broader sense, to all who fund public health, that is, the public.

But what I initially regarded as a mistake by the White House and a major problem for public health turned out fine for reasons I had not anticipated. George Lundberg was the editor of *JAMA* from 1982 to 1999. A pathologist by training, Lundberg was one of those people interested in everything. To be editor of a journal that encompassed all things medical and beyond was a great job fit. Lundberg visited the CDC as part of his information gathering, and when he heard about the White House decision to stop free *MMWR* distribution, he offered to publish the newsletter's contents as a part of *JAMA*. Suddenly, the *MMWR*'s circulation went far beyond the original mailing and could be found in every medical library and in most physicians' offices. It was an important marriage of public health and clinical medicine.

The *MMWR* is only one form of communication for the CDC. Dialogue with workers in the field, articles published in the scientific literature, and employee interviews by journals, newspapers, radio, and television to explain findings are all important. These activities are augmented by countless speeches at countless meetings by hundreds of CDC workers to provide real-time information and dialogue.

A component of responsiveness is providing accurate information to the press (and now, of course, social and other online media). Many organizations attempt to control, at a central point, information released to the press. We took a different approach and told the staff we were comfortable with anyone's talking to the press. We wanted the most knowledgeable people providing the information rather than a spokesperson providing information from talking points. But we had one caveat: tell us what you said so that we don't contradict you. People will talk off the record if this approach isn't used; this way, the front office knew what was being said. We never once got into trouble because of this open approach.

Direct Public Health Response

Daily public health activities are the responsibility of local health departments. Vaccinations, collection of water samples, inspection of restaurants, investigations of outbreaks, and the like are all activities of state, county, and city health departments.

However, the CDC becomes involved as a resource and a provider of skills, consultation, and supplies. For example, the announcement in April 1955 that the Salk vaccine protected against polio led to a federal program to provide polio vaccine to all children in the United States. New vaccines were added to that program, and today it is a massive program that covers many vaccines provided through the CDC to state and local health departments. A part of accepting the vaccine is an agreement on how the vaccine will be used, age groups to receive the vaccine, and standards and evaluations of the immunization program. While the CDC does not routinely administer vaccines, it is heavily involved in the entire immunization program and maintains records on cases of vaccine-preventable diseases. It also provides federal employees to assist states in executing programs, and it offers help in investigating outbreaks of these diseases.

The same is true for many conditions. Investigators are assigned for sexually transmitted diseases, tuberculosis control, environmental health programs, occupational health, and, increasingly, for chronic diseases. Although these investigators are federal employees, they are supervised by state and local health departments. In recent years, the CDC has also assigned hundreds of workers to foreign countries to assist in executing programs for malaria, AIDS, immunization, and training in epidemiology or laboratory sciences.

Speeches

I found myself expected to give many speeches a week, at times two or more a day, and made the unhappy discovery that I could not read a speech prepared by someone else. If I had not written it, I did not understand it well enough to actually give it.

Yet there is scarcely time to write speeches amid the numerous expectations of the CDC director. I used to say that every week felt like test week in medical school with more information than can be easily digested. I had to find an efficient way to prepare talks. And so I developed a system of preparing with the minimum effort possible. I would have a separate file for each speech scheduled over the next few months, and I would go through the files for a half-hour, early each morning. It became an efficient way to update thoughts on multiple subjects. Additional benefits were that this process helped to clarify what I needed to know to convey an idea to an audience, caused me to reach out to the experts in the field, and provided both contact with employees throughout the CDC and a better understanding of what they were doing. So speeches became a way to convey information to others but also (following the medical school test week comparison) forced me to study what was likely to appear on the next test.

On my retirement, I found my files actually contain thousands of speeches. I also found that the market for old speeches is limited (see sidebar).

The Hazards of Giving Speeches

Three stories about my speechmaking always make me smile. The first: Every speaker has a nightmare story of following an exceptional speaker. I wrote this account shortly after my own experience:

> I was asked to speak at the thirtieth anniversary of the Indian Health Service. I did a fair amount of research and was impressed by the reduction in infant mortality and the improvement of other indices in its thirty-year history. Indeed, I became more excited about the results in light of no attempt to change the basic living patterns, a basic tenet of many overseas development programs. Even though the Navajo dwellings, or hogans, were still common and despite the lack of running water or bathrooms, the health indices were improving. There were important lessons here for the developing world.
>
> I traveled to Aberdeen, South Dakota, and met up with the Weltys, both physicians, before my talk. They had arranged for my invitation to be on the program. The turnout was good, and I looked forward to speaking.
>
> The speaker preceding me was William Mervin "Billy" Mills. Mr. Mills was a Sioux hero, who had won a gold medal in the 1964 Olympics in Tokyo, running the 10,000-meter race, the only American who had ever won that event at the Olympics. And what a speaker he was. He showed the actual film clips of his race. Of course, everyone knew, even before he started speaking, that he had won, but as the film went on, he narrated his thoughts as the race was progressing. This included the thoughts he had of dropping out and the decision to take the lead for one lap and then drop out. He could always use an excuse of a twisted ankle. He thought he would feel OK about that decision as he would show what he could do, but he would not have to do it beyond a lap. The Sioux Nation would be proud that he led the world for that one lap. But as he took the lead, giving a great fright to the other runners, he found that he felt fine and that he had enough energy to do it for another lap. He kept playing that game in his mind, lap after lap. He could feel fine dropping out at the completion of the next lap. He had a strong desire to show what a Native American could do. He had pride

in his heritage . . . a pride that increasingly made it impossible to give up. But he also had pain that was eating away at his resolve, and he described the depths of determination that countered the pain.

The audience was beginning to cheer, and they were on their feet as the film showed the end of the race. They could not be restrained. They continued to clap and cheer, and the moderator had trouble regaining order.

But at last the restless crowd was utterly spent and began to contain their enthusiasm and find their seats. Slowly the noise decreased. When all excess energy had been exhausted, the moderator said, "And now to review the last 30 years of Indian health care . . ."

The second speech-related story concerned a lecture I was to give at Johns Hopkins. I checked into the hotel the night before and worked on notes for the talk. When I was almost finished, I went to the lobby bar, ordered a beer, and continued to review my notes.

A talkative man took a seat near me, ordered a drink, and began asking questions, *Where are you from? How long have you been here? When will you go home?* I was polite but continued to work on my notes. He suddenly asked me, "Has anyone ever told you that you have a great personality?" I said, "No." He responded, "Well, there is a reason." But he continued and said, "I didn't come here to talk to you anyway. I came to seduce the piano player." With that he left and went across the room to the piano, where a young woman was playing. I returned to my notes and would have forgotten the episode except that he returned after ten minutes and said, "You are never going to believe this. She has a worse personality than you have."

Finally, a story from a CDC staff meeting, when I was a director, that I am afraid has become legendary. Part of internal communications is to make sure that everyone knows what is going on. Before e-mail became ubiquitous, staff meetings were the principal way of making certain that everyone in a particular office had the same information, so such meetings were frequent. However, I realized the difficulty of keeping the meetings short and informative when Don Berreth, director of the Information Office, once fell asleep in a staff meeting and later said in his defense, "The only ones not sleeping were the ones not listening."

Investigations

The key to public health is appropriate response. That is more than analysis, communication, and support of the daily activities of state and local health departments. It often involves investigations or additional research. Much response is in the form of consulting. States, counties, cities, and foreign countries ask the CDC for advice on how to respond to a problem and then another group conducts the actual response.

Sometimes the request is more formal, for example, a state asking for assistance. In general, the federal government cannot conduct an investigation in a state without an invitation. In practice, this is usually easily arranged because the relationship between the CDC and state and local health departments is so close. In these cases, the appropriate CDC person summarizes the request, usually in less than a one-page report of what is known at that moment, who made the request, when and how the request was conveyed, and how the CDC responded. This is classified as the "EPI 1" document. When the investigation is completed, an "EPI 2" is written to summarize what was done, what was found, and the remedial action taken.

Dozens of such formal investigations are conducted each year, many by current EIS officers together with other CDC staff. In addition, EIS officers assigned to the field do many investigations within their area of assignment that are not formally documented at the CDC, as these officers are working under the supervision of the local health department. The agreement with states is that the officers can be withdrawn for short periods, after discussion with the state health department, for investigations undertaken by CDC headquarters.

In addition, the CDC has many officers assigned to positions in other countries, some through the WHO and some directly with agreements between governments.

The key message is that there should always be a response, just as one would expect in clinical medicine. There are times, as with individual patients, in which the response is watchful waiting, but even that is a response.

Finally, there are long-term efforts with the states to plan for the overall improvement of the public's health. In the 1970s and 1980s, a great deal of time was spent developing standards for every aspect of public health. I frequently observed that baseball had better standards and rules than public health. Baseball fans knew the standards and rules, and daily newspaper accounts would mention them in baseball stories. Pitchers were traded on the basis of not meeting a standard. Games were lost because a rule had been violated. And baseball is only a game. Why couldn't public health be that organized?

In 1978, the Public Health Service decided it was time to develop objectives for the health of the public, in addition to standards. Drs. Julius Richmond and Michael McGinnis were prime movers in the Public Health Service. Representatives from around the country were assembled to begin the process of determining health objectives for the year 1990. The first meeting was held at Emory University in Atlanta, Georgia, followed the next day by a meeting at the CDC. Experts in multiple areas developed more than 200 health objectives. The process is common now and has led to global health and development goals.

The process was so new in 1978 that many of our objectives were unrealistic. But in some ways that did not matter because the important result was that a process had been developed that has continued ever since, and that process continues to get better.

When these objectives were reviewed in 1990, approximately half had been realized, and a quarter had not, although progress was real in most areas. Interestingly, a quarter of the objectives were not even measurable because the measurement tools had proven deficient. But again, that fact served to provide a research agenda on how to improve the system.

This domestic effort to suggest objectives in health led to a similar global effort in 1988. Rafe Henderson, formerly a CDC smallpox worker in West Africa, was now director of the Expanded Program on Immunization at WHO. In March 1988, at a polio meeting in Talloires, France, hosted by the Task Force for Child Survival, he presented a paper on objectives for global child health.

This was a forerunner of the Millennium Development Goals (MDGs) developed by the United Nations. The MDGs will have similar frustrations because of targets not reached or measurement difficulties that hinder evaluation. But the result will be the same as for the health objectives for the nation: they will provide a process, transparency, and a system for future improvements.

chapter 15

VACCINES

The Foundation of Public Health

As Alex Langmuir briefed us on the new oral polio vaccine in the summer of 1962, the future was hidden from me. It would take years for me to appreciate how important vaccines would be in my life. My mother had left me the baby book she bought before my birth in early 1936. It lists only two vaccines to be given to me, diphtheria toxoid and smallpox vaccine. That number, as of this writing, has increased to eighteen routinely given and another dozen for use under special circumstances or for those going to other countries to live or travel.

It has gradually become apparent that vaccines are the foundation of public health. Unlike antibiotics, which must be administered each time a person has an infection and which frequently lose effectiveness against certain organisms, vaccines often provide lifetime protection without developing resistance. Vaccines have become so effective that parents often forget the power of the preventable illness because it is rarely seen, and they become lax or even hostile to the notion of vaccinating their children.

The concept behind vaccines is to fool the immune system. In some cases, a living organism, basically harmless for most but not all people, is introduced into the body, and the immune system develops antibodies to fight that organism. But the harmless organism is so close to a pathogen that causes problems that the person now has immunity to the dangerous one.

Early Vaccines

The first such vaccine was for smallpox. It required no manipulation in the laboratory. Instead, Edward Jenner, practicing medicine in Berkeley, England, observed that milkmaids were protected against smallpox if they had a minor infection on their hands caused by a virus acquired from the teats of cows. Cows would have lesions on their udders and teats, due to a virus later called cowpox virus, but they were not otherwise sick. Milkmaids would get lesions on their hands but no general illness. Yet they were protected against smallpox. This protection was a huge benefit, derived from a natural development and the power of keen observation. Apparently, some milkmaids recognized this, and one even told Jenner she was protected against smallpox because of the lesions on her hand.

Jenner, over the period of a dozen years, observed the experiences of the milkmaids during smallpox outbreaks until he was sure the observation was correct. On May 14, 1796, Jenner was ready to apply his theory, based on those observations. He took material from the hand lesion of milkmaid Sarah Nelmes and, cutting into the skin of 8-year-old James Phipps, he inserted the pus from the cowpox lesion. James developed a fever and recovered. Some weeks later, Jenner inoculated the boy with material from a smallpox patient's pustules. James did not develop smallpox. The cowpox had protected him. We are pleased with the safeguards we have today with ethics committees overseeing such experiments, but we also cannot help but be pleased that Jenner's work presented public health with the first real tool that could be used to prevent disease. From that perspective, May 14, 1796, was the birth date of modern public health.

Building on this first observation, science developed vaccines by using the actual organisms but modifying them so that they would still stimulate the production of antibodies but would not cause disease. In 1937, a scientist working at the Rockefeller Foundation did just that with a strain of the virus causing yellow fever.

Yellow fever viruses cause a severe illness characterized by fever, chills, nausea, muscle pain, and oftentimes liver involvement and jaundice—hence, the name. Death is common. Even today, with a safe and effective vaccine, the WHO estimates that approximately 30,000 people die of yellow fever each year.

Deaths are especially common in populations not previously exposed to the virus. The early history of Europeans in West and Central Africa is replete with reports of very high death rates from yellow fever in explorers, military troops, missionaries, and traders. While Africa was often referred to as the "white man's grave," what is often missed is that it was also the "black man's grave." Local populations might seem to fair well during a yellow fever epidemic, but that was because of a high price of death and illness in childhood that left survivors relatively immune to the disease.

Yellow fever viruses are transmitted by the bite of a mosquito, usually *Aedes aegypti*. The viruses apparently traveled from primates to humans in Central Africa, from there to West Africa, and finally to the Americas with the slave trade. While we think of it as a tropical disease, New York City had an outbreak in 1668. An outbreak in Philadelphia in 1793 led to thousands of deaths and the flight of George Washington and the national government from the then-capital of the United States.

The anxiety can be imagined. No one knew what caused the disease or how it spread; therefore, outbreaks led to panic as people tried to flee the area of the first cases. Some towns would lose a quarter of their population. The social disruption is evident from an outbreak in Memphis in 1878, when people boarded a steamship to head north in hopes of avoiding the outbreak, only to be refused permission to disembark because areas north of Memphis feared the disease. The passengers were trapped on the boat for several months before they could disembark.

Construction of the Panama Canal started in January 1881 but was abandoned, partly because of the high death rates from yellow fever.

But the mysteries of the disease were about to yield to science. Carlos Finlay, a Cuban physician, proposed in the early 1880s that mosquitoes might transmit the disease. (Sixteen years later, Sir Ronald Ross, working in India, would discover the role of mosquitoes in the spread of malaria.) Yellow fever was so devastating in the Spanish American War that the United States developed a team, headed by Walter Reed, to research the problem. The team confirmed Finlay's belief that mosquitoes were an essential ingredient in the transmission of yellow fever from person to person.

At last there was an explanation, and mosquito control now made it possible to actually complete the Panama Canal. (It also allowed Wade Hampton Frost and his team to control an outbreak of yellow fever in New Orleans, even before the first frost killed the mosquitoes.)

In the early twentieth century, the Rockefeller Foundation became interested in the problem, and after World War I the foundation expanded yellow fever work to Africa with a laboratory near Lagos, Nigeria. It was to be both productive and tragic. One member of the group, Adrian Stokes, a pathology professor from London, was the first victim of yellow fever. The next was Hideyo Noguchi, a physician from Japan who worked at the Rocke-feller Institute. His autopsy was performed by William Young, who also died of yellow fever. Global health work was high risk at that time. But they did not give up.

Then a series of breakthroughs permitted the isolation of a virus and transport of that virus in a frozen state to New York. Work at the Rockefeller Institute with cell cultures led to the development of the 17D yellow fever vaccine by Theiler and Haagen. Theiler, from South Africa, hired in 1930 from Harvard by the Rockefeller Foundation, received a Nobel Prize in 1951 for his work.

The vaccine is so protective that many thought yellow fever eradication would be a reasonable undertaking. The WHO supported such a program, only to find that primates are also infected with the virus. Indeed, workers and hunters in the forests are often the link between primate transmission and human outbreaks. Short of immunizing primates (not impossible if oral vaccines are developed that could be included in food baits of various kinds), eradication is not possible, and efforts are now focused on protect-ing populations living in yellow fever-endemic areas, as well as travelers to those areas.

For reasons not totally clear, Asia has been spared from the virus. Public health workers are always concerned that a traveler could introduce the virus and that, because the appropriate mosquitoes are already in Asia, a mas-sive outbreak could ensue. For that reason, Asian countries are very strict about travelers showing proof of vaccination. It takes no special insight to predict that, at some time in the future, yellow fever will spread to Asia.

The vaccine inventory now contains many other live vaccines that have been modified to avoid disease. They are capable of multiplying in the per-son receiving the vaccine so that the immune system develops antibodies. Measles, mumps, and rubella (MMR) vaccines are examples of such live vaccines.

Polio Vaccine

Another category of vaccines includes organisms that have been killed so that they cannot cause the disease, and yet the immune system recog-nizes them as a threat and develops antibodies to fight them as if they were live invaders.

The Salk vaccine, is an example. Physicians Tom Weller, John Enders, and Fred Robbins were working on improving the ability to identify and grow viruses in the laboratory. It was while working on techniques to grow chickenpox viruses in cell cultures, in 1949, that Tom Weller found that poliovirus would replicate in the culture materials he was attempting to develop for chickenpox virus. He immediately shifted his focus to polioviruses, and the team was able to grow unlimited quantities of the virus in the lab.

The ability to grow large quantities of the poliovirus allowed Jonas Salk to develop a vaccine based on killing the virus and inoculating the killed virus. Within three years, he had a vaccine shown to be effective in producing antibodies in a small study. But would it protect against polio? Salk was not convinced that a field trial was even necessary. He was certain that the ability of the vaccine to produce antibodies was proof that it would protect against polio disease. In his mind, it would be immoral to have a control group, who would remain unvaccinated. But his mentor, Thomas Francis, the first person to isolate an influenza virus, simply said, "That is not the way science works." Francis agreed to organize the field trial in 1953, and in two years, with the help of 1.8 million children, countless volunteers, and superb organization, Thomas Francis had an answer.

Yet a third type of vaccine is in common use. For some illnesses, the organism does not cause the illness but rather a toxin produced by the organism, for example, tetanus. Acquiring a tetanus spore does not automatically lead to illness. However, when the tetanus organism produces a toxin, tetanospasmin, which affects the nerves that lead to muscles, illness results. This neurotoxin causes the muscles to contract, leading to spasms. Often the jaw muscles are affected first (hence, the name *lockjaw*) with life-threatening results when respiratory muscles become involved. This toxin is second only to botulinum in potency, and yet it is totally neutralized by antibodies and therefore disease can be prevented. A vaccine derived from the toxin allows each person to develop his or her own protection, even in the face of an environment loaded with tetanus organisms.

The tetanus vaccine is one of the best vaccines in our arsenal. Attempts to see how long the vaccine provided protection led to studies in World War II veterans who developed tetanus over the years after the war. In most cases, it was found that the veterans, for various reasons, had not actually received the vaccine; in fact, some admitted to having others receive the vaccine for them because they were so adverse to needle sticks.

Gradually, various vaccines became routine. However, vaccines such as smallpox vaccine, diphtheria toxoid, tetanus toxoid, and pertussis vaccine were generally administered by doctors, and the patients paid for those vaccines. They were not purchased by public health programs seeking widespread coverage. This all changed on April 12, 1955.

Today, it is almost impossible to understand the fear that gripped people in the mid-twentieth century as they contemplated polio. The fear was similar to that felt by Africans and Indians in the 1970s for smallpox or Americans in 2014 in the face of Ebola disease. An anthropologist who lived through a smallpox outbreak with the Tiv people of Nigeria said the only comparison that could be understood by those outside the outbreak might be the experience of war.

The fear of polio grew during the first half of the twentieth century. Epidemics were rare until the end of the nineteenth century because children often acquired the viruses in the first year of life, when passive immunity from their mothers allowed the virus to grow in their intestine; maternal immunity prevented the virus from entering the central nervous system (hence, no paralysis). As hygiene improved, the risk of exposure to polio in the first year decreased and children began to acquire the wild virus after they had lost maternal immunity, often upon entering school. Most cases were therefore in young children, and the disease acquired the name *infantile paralysis*. Over time, the virus was no longer ubiquitous and might be introduced to a community only after several years had passed and a group of susceptible children had accumulated. Outbreaks resulted, and the age of patients increased. By midcentury, epidemics during summer months became common, and some of those paralyzed were adolescents and young adults.

In 1952, the United States reported almost 58,000 cases of polio. More than 3,000 of these patients died, and more than 20,000 persons were left with various degrees of paralysis. Scientists were working overtime to find an answer to this problem. Interest was also heightened because of the paralysis of President Franklin Roosevelt. Clearly, everyone was at risk, even the rich such as Roosevelt.

The National Foundation for Infantile Paralysis was established. Eddie Cantor suggested the phrase "The March of Dimes," based on a popular news program shown at theaters called *The March of Time*. Contributions of dimes flowed into the White House, and research efforts were accelerated.

Jonas Salk was one scientist funded by the organization, and he established that three types of the virus existed. But then he benefited from the breakthrough by John Enders, Tom Weller, and Fred Robbins, when they demonstrated that the virus could grow under laboratory conditions. These three later received the Nobel Prize for their findings.

The killed vaccine was soon ready for a field trial, but the logistics would prove difficult. Even in epidemics, only a small percentage of children would show evidence of illness, and even fewer (less than 1 percent) would show the characteristic paralysis; therefore, an enormous study was required to have sufficient numbers of children with paralysis. So Francis, before the age of computers, had to assemble a team of 20,000 medical personnel, 64,000 school personnel, and 220,000 volunteers. With that as a core, he then enrolled 1.8 million schoolchildren into this massive study. It was said that file cabinets lined hallway after hallway at the University of Michigan.

On April 12, 1955, ten years to the day after the death of Franklin D. Roosevelt, Francis faced an overflow audience at Rackham Auditorium, including scientists and noted journalists, such as Edward R. Murrow and Fred Friendly. He summarized the two-year study in four words: "safe, effective and potent." Pandemonium ensued, as reporters tried to get to phones. The next day a grateful nation spontaneously put signs in windows that read, "Thank you, Dr. Salk."

Salk once related to me the story of that day. He said Murrow interviewed him on CBS television and asked, "Who owns the patent on this vaccine?" Salk answered, "Well, the people, I would say. There is no patent. Could you patent the sun?" That night at dinner, Murrow presented Salk with a watch that he wore for the rest of his life. Murrow said, "Young man, today you have lost your anonymity."

It was a great day in public health, and it changed medical history. But in a real sense, a greater day would occur within the week.

A Social Contract

On April 11, 1953, President Eisenhower named Oveta Culp Hobby to be the first secretary of the new Department of Health, Education, and Welfare (HEW). She was an accomplished manager as the head of the Women's Army Corps during World War II. She had made it clear that socialized medicine would not get any support from her.

But now the polio vaccine was declared effective, and people assumed there would be a government plan for its distribution. The public clamored, and President Eisenhower asked Secretary Hobby for a plan.

Secretary Hobby announced that she would seek an appropriation to buy polio vaccine for poor children. Soon, a senator responded by saying that no American children should have to declare themselves poor to be protected from polio, and he would seek an appropriation to provide polio vaccine for all children and pregnant women. *This is the day that vaccines went from only protecting the recipient to a social contract that attempted to protect society.* It was the beginning of a public health immunization program for this country. Three months later, that senator, Senator Lister Hill, introduced bill S. 2501 authorizing the government to buy polio vaccine.

A decade later, President Lyndon Johnson used the same logic of a social contract to commit the United States to the global eradication of smallpox.

The Cutter Incident

Paul Offit has chronicled the tragedy that quickly overtook the joy of that University of Michigan announcement (1). There was a time when Dr. Salk had questioned the need for a field trial. Tommy Francis had overruled that idea, and now everyone was happy that he had. Because within the month, the value of the field trial would become obvious to all.

Only six days after the University of Michigan press conference, on April 18, 1955, Josephine Gottsdanker drove her two children to the pediatrician to get the new vaccine. She had seen Edward R. Murrow's interview with Jonas Salk, and she wanted her children protected. The family went on vacation, but as they returned, on April 26, her daughter complained of a headache. She soon developed paralysis. And, as Offit points out, 40,000 other children also developed symptoms after getting the Salk vaccine; 200 were paralyzed, and 10 died. What was going on? (1).

Alex Langmuir immediately put his officers on the case. Overnight, at the request of the surgeon general, Langmuir developed a national polio surveillance system to detect cases of polio as rapidly as they developed and then to get information on every case. How old were the patients, when did symptoms begin, where and when did they get vaccine, and which manufacturer made the vaccine they received? The polio surveillance system was quickly developed and improved as the outbreak was investigated.

This was the second national surveillance system developed in this country. The first had been instituted five years earlier for malaria; it revealed that malaria had quietly disappeared in this country. We now have dozens of national surveillance systems for many conditions. But it was the polio surveillance system that demonstrated the value and power of aggregate data.

Public health workers toiled around the clock and quickly demonstrated that the postvaccine cases were heavily concentrated in California and Idaho.

A number of companies were producing the vaccine, but Langmuir quickly realized that the people with paralysis had shared one thing. They had received vaccine made by Cutter Laboratories. The Francis field trial had demonstrated both the safety and the effectiveness of the vaccine. This made it possible for Langmuir to provide assurance that vaccines made by other companies were safe to use. Langmuir demonstrated the power of the epidemiologic approach by predicting what the epidemic curve of cases would look like, given the number of doses of Cutter vaccine given, and what the secondary attack rate would be due to new cases resulting from contact with the vaccine-induced case-patients. He was close on both counts. What was the problem? The process for killing the poliovirus was incomplete. Relatively few live viruses survived to make it into the vaccine vial, but it was enough to cause illness in some of the thousands of children receiving vaccine from that company.

The Cutter incident was a vivid reminder of the need for federal regulations on vaccine safety and for oversight to enforce such regulations. It also demonstrated the absolutely crucial need for field trials to establish the safety, efficacy, and potency of vaccines. But from the CDC's perspective, it also demonstrated the need for a federal program to collect and interpret data from the entire country and the need to provide guidance on the use of vaccines. This incident also established the reputation of the EIS.

Polio incidence in the United States declined by more than 95 percent from 1955 until 1961, when the new Sabin oral vaccine was introduced. The Salk vaccine was a killed product (with the exception of that which caused the Cutter incident); by contrast, the Sabin vaccine was a live but attenuated virus that could be given orally with a sugar cube. The vaccine virus would then multiply in the intestine of the recipient. Despite the small risks of acquiring polio from the oral vaccine, it was adopted in the United States because of its ease of administration. It was also believed that it had the benefit of providing immunity in the intestine. This would reduce transmission of the wild virus if acquired by children who had received the oral vaccine. This attribute of oral vaccine was overestimated, but it took years to discover that the Salk vaccine also provided considerable intestinal immunity, although slightly less than the oral Sabin vaccine.

In 1979, the United States experienced its last polio outbreak. Polio cases occurred in the unimmunized Amish communities in Pennsylvania. Several things were significant about this outbreak. Not only was it the last outbreak in the United States but also it was the first time CDC scientists were able to fingerprint a poliovirus. They were able to show that a single strain of wild poliovirus was responsible for all the cases. Second, as the outbreak spread to other Amish communities in other states, it was possible to show that only one strain was still involved. Third, polio cases were not identified outside the Amish community, providing some reassurance that it was not exceptionally easy for the virus to reestablish after it had disappeared from a geographic area. Fourth, it was possible to trace the virus backward; it had been introduced from within a religious community in Canada, traveling there from a religious community in the Netherlands, which had received the virus from the Middle East. But finally, and of great importance, the Amish taught an important lesson regarding the social contract of vaccines. For religious reasons, they had not immunized their children. When they realized their children presented a risk to non-Amish children, they immediately agreed to a polio immunization campaign.

This last lesson continues to reverberate decades later. As polio, measles, and whooping cough cases declined, parents lost their fear of the diseases. Soon they concentrated on only one side of the equation, the risk of the vaccine. All vaccines have some inherent risks, although these have declined as the vaccines have gotten purer and better over the years. Nonetheless, enough parents have decided against immunization to increase once again the risk of the diseases. In 1989 and 1990, the United States suffered thousands of cases of measles and dozens of resulting deaths.

Improving the National Immunization Program

In 1977, President Jimmy Carter was inaugurated. Early in his tenure, the Carters invited Senator Dale Bumpers and his wife Betty for dinner at the White House. The two wives had become friends when both were First Ladies, Mrs. Carter in Georgia and Mrs. Bumpers in Arkansas. They shared many interests but one was the need to protect more children with the vaccines that were becoming increasingly available. Now at the dinner table, the two women became excited over the prospect of improving the immunization status of children throughout the country.

The next morning, President Carter called his new secretary of HEW, Joseph Califano, to discuss what it would take to improve the national immunization program. Secretary Califano called me, not to discuss what it would take but rather to say we were going to do it. He suggested we set a goal of 90 percent coverage with childhood vaccines by a child's entry into school.

I, in turn, went to Don Millar, the head of the CDC Immunization Program, and asked him what it would take to reach 90 percent immunization levels? Don had considerable experience with immunization and the barriers to good programs, both domestically and internationally, as head of the Smallpox Eradication/Measles Control Program in West and Central Africa. He had worked in the polio programs in which the Sabin live polio vaccine was given on special Sunday clinics. Even our best, concentrated efforts rarely saw immunization rates exceed 90 percent. His response to the 90 percent goal was typically concise and well reasoned. He said, "I would not like to see that in my job description!" But he agreed that a 90 percent target should be attempted, and the next day it was in his job description.

In typical Millarian fashion, Don rose to the occasion, energizing immunization programs around the country to acquire more staff, increase coverage targets, involve education departments and PTA programs, and increase the news coverage on the diseases and the immunization programs. Everything advanced. The public health structure continued to improve management, evaluation, surveillance, and outcomes. States without school-entry requirements worked on ways to involve political leaders. Only seventeen states had school-entry immunization requirements, but over the next few years, activists were able to get politicians to pass such requirements in all states. Education leaders joined the coalition, and over time, the figures inched up more than 90 percent and then even to the 95 percent level. Don had incredibly gifted immunization leaders. Physicians Alan Hinman, Walt Orenstein, Steve Cochi, and others were zealots. They understood the benefits of protecting children with vaccines, and they wanted every child to enjoy that benefit.

Success led to additional objectives. One was to exceed 95 percent; a second was to achieve that percentage by age 2, rather than wait for school entry. And a third objective seemed almost beyond our reach: Could we actually interrupt measles transmission in the United States?

Interrupting Measles Transmission

The last objective resulted in a lively debate. Measles is so easily transmitted that it almost seems mysterious. Introduce one child with measles into a room of susceptible children, and more than 75 percent are likely to become ill after one incubation period. Some scientists argued that to even declare such an objective would lead to ridicule and that we would hurt the reputation of the CDC by failing such a target, and failure would be inevitable.

When Dave Sencer suggested a measles eradication goal some years earlier, many did indeed ridicule the idea. Others maintained, more persuasively, that we would never understand the actual barriers to interrupting the transmission of this virus unless we sought the ultimate objective, stopping its spread. After considered deliberation, we decided to interrupt measles transmission in the United States.

We reserved a thirty-minute segment each week to review what we had achieved and what we had learned about measles. Like the peeling of an onion, each week brought a new problem, not fully understood in the past, but each week also brought possible solutions. That was the payoff of this weekly investment of time by an array of CDC talent. For all of our worry, we never discovered a problem that did not have an eventual solution.

The first problem was the realization that military recruits were a source of measles virus spread. As new recruits went on their first home leave, they often took the virus back to their homes. The military solved this with a single change. From then on, they would immunize all new recruits, regardless of their history of measles disease or measles immunization. Within the first year, the problem of the military as a source of civilian infections was identified and totally resolved.

Next, the immunization program discovered that transmission was occurring from preschool programs, which had not been included in the school-entry requirements. States then methodically changed their requirements to include preschool programs. This was a multiyear project.

Each solution made another problem more visible. Soon, for example, we found that transmission was occurring in college and postgraduate programs. But the problems were getting smaller and more discrete. An outbreak of measles resulted from a wrestling match; thus, it became clear that close contact gives the measles virus an added chance to spread. A wedding involving two important Romany families held in Spokane, Washington, drew families from around the country, and the virus spread as they returned home. Each problem identified a group requiring special attention.

A baffling outbreak involved children who had visited Disneyland. The affected children had attended on different days, leading us to believe that the index case-patient must actually work at the park. (While this was undoubtedly true, the index case-patient was not identified.) It is possible to work while sick with measles, if you are not too ill. And you can avoid identification if you are dressed as a Disney character.

But soon we realized that such outbreaks had masked our biggest, remaining risk: imported cases. These constituted the core of the remaining measles problem. The United States was experiencing, on average, two importations of measles a week from other countries—a fact that had always been obscured by indigenous transmission.

With this information, the Pan American Health Organization continued to improve measles immunization programs in the Americas. Soon we went weeks without a case. The United States reached the point that measles was no longer accepted as a childhood disease, and the presence of cases became front-page news. It took five years of effort to stop endemic transmission of measles in the United States, but for a quarter of a century, all measles cases in this country have been the result of importation. Choosing the ultimate objective was the only way to make this possible.

In summary, vaccine-preventable deaths have drastically declined in the United States, thanks to a national immunization program that involves politicians and government and health workers at every point from national, state, county, and city levels. It is a grand coalition of public and private organizations. This has been a wonderfully successful program for the country.

There are other vaccine success stories. These include the reduction of pneumonia and meningitis when *Haemophilus influenzae* vaccine was introduced. And the elimination of the dreaded congenital rubella syndrome in newborns, when rubella vaccine, given to enough children, halted transmission of the virus in this country. The United States has also been blessed by the reduction of deaths from influenza and pneumonia in the young and in the elderly.

The development of an anticancer vaccine against human papillomavirus (HPV) presents another opportunity to seek an ultimate solution. This virus is often silent after acquisition through sexual contact but can later cause cancer in both men and women. The most prevalent of these cancers is cancer of the cervix. As a result, many programs have focused on girls and young women before they become sexually active. However, the real challenge is to stop transmission of the virus, and, as with measles, our objective should be breaking virus transmission and nothing less. The combination of an HPV vaccine and early screening for carcinoma of the cervix means that there should never be another death from cervical cancer in this country.

A View of Vaccine History

It was at the 1995 memorial service for Dr. Jonas Salk, at the Salk Institute in San Diego, that I developed a startling mental picture of the entire history of immunization programs. For the occasion, Dr. Charles Merieux had traveled from France, and he reviewed the history of immunizations. He talked about the movement from eighteenth-century England and Edward Jenner, to nineteenth-century France and Louis Pasteur and then to twentieth-century America and Jonas Salk.

I immediately thought about my visit to the home of Dr. Merieux in France, where he showed me a picture on his wall. He said, "That is my father, working in the lab. And the man standing next to him is Dr. Louis Pasteur!" That moment is riveted in my mind because it was Louis Pasteur, while on a visit to London, who changed our nomenclature. He noted, in a speech, that the word *vaccine* refers specifically to the virus used to protect against smallpox, namely vaccinia virus, and that the word *vaccination* refers to the inoculation of vaccinia virus. However, Pasteur suggested that from this time forth, we could honor Edward Jenner by referring to all immunizing agents as vaccines and the application of those agents as vaccinations. With that, I could visualize the entire history from Jenner to Pasteur to Merieux and now Salk.

Our Debt to Hilleman

But there is yet another hero who must be recognized. Maurice Hilleman was born on a ranch in Montana. His twin sister died at birth, and his mother died two days later. Because of lack of money, Hilleman almost went to work after high school, without the chance of going to college. But a brother continued to urge him to find a way, and eventually he made it through college, graduating first in his class. He then received a PhD from the University of Chicago, where he demonstrated that *Chlamydia* organisms were not viruses, as thought, but rather bacteria. He was already thinking beyond the horizons of his teachers.

Why mention him here? I gave two Maurice Hilleman lectures during his lifetime, and he attended both of them. In the first, I referred to him as the Louis Pasteur of our time. In the second, I corrected myself. Hilleman was in a class by himself, exceeding any vaccine developer the world has ever seen. Over half of the vaccines reaching our children today either came out of his mind directly or were altered in some way by his ideas. He was a complex and compelling genius.

He was an exceedingly capable scientist, able to see things denied to others. He was an obsessive worker, who expected his coworkers to meet his standards. He was a difficult man to work with; he kept a row of "shrunken heads" in his office (constructed by his children) to represent the people he had fired. He was coarse and vulgar and could use profanity with as much ingenuity and directness as he used science. Roy Vagelos, former CEO of Merck, confirmed that Hilleman had failed the compulsory "charm school" course required of Merck supervisors. But his subordinates loved him. He got the most out of them but only because they were willing to give it to a man who outworked everyone.

He developed a vaccine against Japanese B encephalitis, and a vaccine against the Hong Kong flu. He went on to develop more than three dozen vaccines for humans and animals. Although his modesty would not allow him to put his name on a vaccine (such as the Salk vaccine or the Sabin vaccine), he did allow the mumps vaccine to be named the Jeryl Lynn strain after his daughter, from whom he isolated the virus. (He was awakened during the night because she had pain in her jaw. He immediately drove to his lab for equipment and returned to successfully culture the mumps virus for the first time.)

Hilleman developed the MMR vaccine. It is given to millions of children every month. A billion children vaccinated against measles in recent years make it possible to contemplate measles eradication in the world.

Hilleman also developed a hepatitis B vaccine. In many countries, this virus, acquired early in life, leads to liver cancer in adults. In some countries, it is the leading cause of death from cancer; therefore, it is a significant problem. Hilleman not only developed a vaccine but also originally surprised everyone by preparing the vaccine from the blood serum of gay men. He treated it with pepsin, urea, and formaldehyde.

The products of Hilleman's mind have entered and changed the immune systems of the majority of the world's population. It is almost beyond comprehension what this one person has meant for global health. And one remains troubled by how close he came to dying at birth like his twin sister, or how close he came to not continuing his education beyond high school. And one also thinks about his vaccines keeping other geniuses from dying in childhood.

After Hilleman's death, at age 85, Ralph Nader wrote, "Yet almost no one knew about him, saw him on television, or read about him in newspapers or magazines. His anonymity, in comparison with Madonna, Michael Jackson, Jose Canseco, or an assortment of grade-B actors, tells something about our society's and media's concept of celebrity; much less of the heroic" (2).

But we knew him well at the CDC.

The Task Force for Child Survival

In late 1983, Jonas Salk and Robert McNamara talked with Jim Grant, head of UNICEF, to discuss how the improvements in the US Immunization Program could benefit immunization programs around the world. Their inquiries led to a meeting at the Rockefeller Center in Bellagio, Italy, in March 1984. The meeting included the directors of UNICEF, WHO, the United Nations Development Programme (UNDP), the World Bank, and USAID, among others. Rafe Henderson, who had been seconded from the CDC to develop the Expanded Program on Immunization at the WHO, also attended (3).

The meeting led to the development of a Task Force for Child Survival, headquartered in Atlanta and largely staffed by former CDC employees. The Task Force held quarterly meetings with the key representatives of UNICEF, WHO, UNDP, the World Bank, and the Rockefeller Foundation. This small group quickly agreed on steps to improve coordination to improve global immunization. More than that, it gave donors confidence that a global approach was being developed rather than multiple agencies working independently.*

Robert McNamara had argued that $100 million in new immunization money would change the world of immunizations. Attendees at the Bellagio meeting argued that could not happen without taking money from other global health programs. But they were wrong. Confidence in a global approach led to new resources, and Italy alone gave $100 million for immunization programs in Africa. They were so impressed with plans that they increased the gift to $120 million. UNICEF and WHO coordinated in new ways, working together in countries, putting out joint publications on evaluating programs and forming partnerships on research to improve efficiency and to present a single voice to countries. However, they could not agree on a name for the program. While the WHO referred to the program as the Expanded Program on Immunization, UNICEF continued to call it Universal Childhood Immunization. But it mattered not. There was unity of purpose, and immunization levels improved. Rafe Henderson always attended the quarterly meetings, representing the WHO; UNICEF would send its top immunization person, but often times Jim Grant himself would attend.

*The story of the impact on global health that this small group grew to have is told in my upcoming book on the history of the Task Force for Child Survival.

For six years, the Task Force met quarterly and approximately every eighteen months would have a larger meeting to include dozens of persons and groups involved in global immunization efforts. Each meeting was able to report on increasing levels of immunization, more coordination between agencies, tighter country programs, and growing excitement over the protection of children with vaccines. With increasing confidence, the group added oral rehydration therapy, micronutrient additions to the immunization program, child health programs of various kinds, and even family planning. It proved that there is a place for collaboration among groups assisting national and global efforts.

The Summit for Children

On September 30, 1990, the United Nations had a one-day "Summit for Children." The program was the product of Jim Grant's enthusiasm and included seventy-one heads of state, to that point the largest gathering of heads of state the world had ever seen. Children in national dress escorted heads of state to their seats.

The heads of state were permitted five minutes to comment on what they had done and what they planned to do to improve child health in their countries. I watched from the audience as peer pressure increased the leaders' promises during the day. Jim Grant declared that immunization levels had improved from about 15 percent six years earlier to the point that 80 percent of children were now receiving at least some of the childhood immunizations. He said this was the greatest peacetime effort the world had ever seen.

A grand coalition such as this requires that heads of agencies are committed. When Jim Grant died and Halfdan Mahler retired as head of the WHO, keeping the same level of commitment was no longer possible. The new director of UNICEF, Carol Bellamy, pursued other objectives and reduced the immunization budget. The new WHO director, the physician Hiroshi Nakajima, found collaboration with other agencies very difficult. The Task Force played a diminished role. Through the 1990s, immunization rates continued to stagnate, and the global coalition that had been so successful through the 1980s was disintegrating. The Task Force for Child Survival became the Task Force for Global Health, and under the leadership of Dr. Mark Rosenberg, it has become one of the most successful nonprofit agencies in the world as it directs products worth billions of dollars each year to neglected diseases of poor countries. In 2016, the Task Force was awarded the Hilton Humanitarian Award that not only acknowledged the Task Force's impact but also was accompanied by a $2 million award to enhance its activities.

A New Global Coalition

In 1998, the World Bank initiated meetings to revitalize the global immunization program, and, in November 1999, the Bill & Melinda Gates Foundation brought life back into the idea of a coalition with the formation of the Global Alliance for Vaccines and Immunization (GAVI). But the alliance went far beyond the modest objectives of the Task Force of 1984. With a pledge of $750 million over five years, the foundation wanted to improve the capacity to deliver vaccines, but it also wanted to add the lifesaving vaccines that were more expensive and had eluded the global community.

The global health community remained somewhat skeptical of the staying power of the foundation, and the matching grants expected early on were not materializing, despite the solid leadership of Tore Godal, the gifted global health worker from Norway, who had spent years working in the WHO and was now heading GAVI. Four years into the program, the Gates Foundation announced that it would renew its pledge for an additional five years. Immediately, Norway and the United Kingdom announced that they would make contributions. A new era in global immunization had arrived. And a former CDC and Task Force employee, Seth Berkley, became the second director of GAVI.

Fear of Autism

One of the most discouraging developments in the vaccine field has been the difficulty in maintaining the immunization levels that have been achieved. In part, this reflects the success of the program in reducing the diseases targeted. Parents no longer compare the risks of vaccine to the risk of the disease. Instead, they compare the risk of vaccine to zero because they cannot visualize the disease's risks.

This problem is potentially correctable through education. In the early years of education on the risks associated with tobacco use, smoking rates were high for physicians. Although nicotine is very addictive, education was able to overcome addiction, and soon smoking rates dropped faster for physicians than for other occupations; the lowest smoking rates were seen in thoracic surgeons and pulmonary specialists, who daily saw the price of tobacco. But, interestingly, smoking rates did not go to zero, even in those groups. Nicotine addiction is powerful.

Education is also the approach required for vaccines. Pediatricians have been in the forefront of the effort to educate parents because they have seen the ravages of the diseases. But even some pediatricians are against immunization. Education is important but not sufficient.

In addition to education, laws and conventions are necessary to protect the largest numbers possible. School-entry requirements, military regulations, and national quarantine regulations all help immensely.

For more than thirty-five years, the custom has been to require consent for immunization. The reason is to make it clear that the parent recognizes the inherent complications of immunizations. It is now proving necessary to also contemplate informed consent from parents who decline immunization for their children. Such parents may need to demonstrate that their declination is truly informed and not simply a lack of knowledge or an antigovernment bias that leads them to accept undue risks for their children. Reminding new parents that their child avoided congenital rubella syndrome because other children had been immunized against rubella is important in explaining the social contract we have to protect our children and other children.

In the midst of all the positive actions that have improved child health, one of the most devastating negative stories concerns a physician from England, Andrew Wakefield, who published an article in the *Lancet* based on twelve children. He raised the question of whether MMR vaccine might be responsible for the increased incidence of autism. The fear of autism is so great that many parents began to refuse vaccinations.

Major studies were undertaken in response to this allegation, and all showed no increase in autism incidence in children who had received the vaccine as compared to those who had not received it. Then concern was raised that thimerosal, an antiseptic containing mercury, might be a problem. Thimerosal had been used in vaccines for many years to prevent bacterial overgrowth in multiple dose vials of vaccine.

Increasingly, single-dose syringes containing vaccines have been used, and they have not required the use of thimerosal. Dropping the use of this agent made no difference in the rates of autism.

As the science became clearer, three facts emerged. First, no evidence existed that vaccines were implicated in the increase in autism. Second, research continued to implicate prenatal factors, especially in the second trimester of pregnancy, rather than postbirth exposures as important in the development of autism. Third, the science could not easily counter the social fear that had now developed around the use of vaccines.

If vaccines had been related to autism, knowing that would have been very important. Therefore, it was important to consider whether any evidence existed to suggest it. However, by the time the question was answered, untold harm had been done as parents heard the preliminary question but not the answer, and many had lost their confidence in vaccines.

On January 6, 2011, the *British Medical Journal* published an article by journalist Brian Deer, who examined the medical records of the twelve children cited in the Andrew Wakefield article (4). His findings:

The paper in *The Lancet* was a case series of 12 child patients; it reported a proposed "new syndrome" of enterocolitis and regressive autism and associated this with MMR as an apparent precipitating event. But in fact:

Three of nine children reported with regressive autism did not have autism diagnosed at all. Only one child clearly had regressive autism;

Despite the paper claiming that all 12 children were previously normal, five had documented pre-existing developmental concerns;

Some children were reported to have experienced first behavioral symptoms within days of MMR, but the records documented these as starting some months after vaccination;

In nine cases, unremarkable colonic histopathology results—noting no or minimal fluctuations in inflammatory cell populations—were changed after a medical school "research review" to "non-specific colitis";

The parents of eight children were reported as blaming MMR, but 11 families made this allegation at the hospital. The exclusion of three allegations—all giving times to onset of problems in months—helped to create the appearance of a 14-day temporal link;

Patients were recruited through anti-MMR campaigners, and the study was commissioned and funded for planned litigation.

In an accompanying editorial (5), *British Medical Journal* editors wrote:

Clear evidence of falsification of data should now close the door on this damaging vaccine scare . . . Who perpetrated this fraud? There is no doubt that it was Wakefield. Is it possible that he was wrong, but not dishonest: that he was so incompetent that he was unable to fairly describe the project, or to report even one of the 12 children's cases accurately? No. A great deal of thought and effort must have gone into drafting the paper to achieve the results he wanted:

the discrepancies all led in one direction; misreporting was gross. Moreover, although the scale of the GMC's 217-day hearing precluded additional charges focused directly on the fraud, the panel found him guilty of dishonesty concerning the study's admissions criteria, its funding by the Legal Aid Board, and his statements about it afterwards.

Perhaps this is too much attention to the negative forces opposing immunization. But when one understands the importance of vaccines to the health of the world, understanding the hollowness of the antivaccination movement seems critical.

Wakefield lost his license to practice in the United Kingdom, but he moved to the United States and has continued talking to parents' groups about the dangers of vaccines. He attempted to sue Deer and the *Sunday Times*, and lost.

Repeatedly, nature is shown to be a formidable foe when it comes to death and disease. But it is discouraging, as with this article by Wakefield, when the enemy turns out to be people seeking fame or profit.

Vaccination efforts will hopefully recover to deliver their promise, but the lesson must be heeded that parents throughout the world are likely to follow the European and American trends. Namely, parents can easily lose interest in certain vaccines when the diseases are no longer prominent.

There will always be charlatans to make public health work more difficult. The media are often more concerned with so-called balance than with truth. Over many decades, we have watched as reports on tobacco have summarized the work of scientists and then, "for balance," the report ends with a quote from the Tobacco Institute, an organization funded by tobacco companies. This makes no logical sense. When confronted, reporters would tell me that this was necessary to show balance. My response was they should clearly label this as the other side of truth. Their ultimate argument was that readers were smart enough to read both sides and see the truth. My contention was that this was unlikely if the reporters themselves were unable to do that.

Likewise with vaccines. Reports by the American Academy of Pediatrics, the Advisory Committee on Immunization Practices, and researchers around the country are often balanced by comments from a publicity-seeking television personality, who has done untold damage by supporting Wakefield and claiming that vaccines cause autism.

Vaccines in the Future

The future of vaccines is exceptionally exciting. Without even entertaining thoughts of science fiction, it is totally predictable that we will eliminate much of the trauma experienced by children because of needles. Increasingly, vaccines will be given orally or transdermally. More vaccines will be combined to reduce the number of medical contacts necessary to protect children.

In addition, the number of vaccines will continue to increase. In seventy-five years, routine vaccines for children in the United States increased from two to eighteen vaccines, and another dozen are given under certain circumstances. My grandchildren will see this number increase to dozens.

Two vaccines are already in the category of anticancer vaccines, protecting against liver cancer and cancer of the cervix. Anticancer vaccines will multiply.

Vaccines will be developed against certain aspects of cardiovascular disease and diabetes, as we understand the role of infectious agents in later chronic diseases. We may even see vaccines that will reduce the desire for alcohol, opiates, and other agents so disruptive to life.

Because of vaccines, the number of diseases eliminated for all time will increase. In addition to smallpox, polio—despite all the social problems encountered with religious and terrorist groups (not to mention US intelligence agencies' misuse of the program in an attempt to identify the house of bin Laden, an act that fueled backlash from terrorist groups, who have killed innocent vaccinators to vent their rage)—will cease to exist. Measles will follow and then the pace may accelerate as the world gains confidence in its ability to understand both the epidemiology of diseases and the sociologic conditions involved in the spread of diseases.

With the improvement of the science base, public health will have formidable challenges in educating people about the benefits of such vaccines and the implications of the social contract in using them.

chapter 16

DO NO HARM

The ethical problems encountered in public health span the spectrum of those seen in clinical medicine, but they have additional ramifications. The oft-repeated admonition First Do No Harm, heard throughout the years of medical training, usually referred to errors of commission. Even when the Institute of Medicine published a book on medical mistakes, it concentrated on such errors (1).

But when Wolf Bulle told me, as I left for Africa in 1965, "You will never forget the people you kill," it caused me to wrestle with that concept.

Errors of Omission

It soon became clear that we will, of course, not know most of the people we kill. Far more people die and suffer because of our errors of omission. The science not used, the science not shared, the vaccines not given, and the prevention not practiced, the Medicaid not expanded, the millions without health insurance, all cause harm but are rarely mentioned or even recognized in the context of First Do No Harm. Because the price of those omissions is usually not seen, it is often discounted.

Medical care today makes it difficult for the busy practitioner to discuss prevention with patients. Most insurance plans do not adequately compensate practitioners for time spent giving prevention advice. A half-century ago, people were worried about socialized medicine without understanding that capitalism would soon take over medical care in the United States. Now profit drives the system, and because of that, it is possible to violate the First Do No Harm dictate repeatedly each day. It is as if we were told in school to do no harm unless money is involved.

We stand embarrassed to spend more per capita on health care than any other country; yet, we cannot match the health outcomes of the top twenty countries around the world. We proudly promote the marketplace as the way to deliver health care without acknowledging that the vast majority of those countries have single-payer systems. Are we interested in promoting the marketplace or promoting health? And isn't the burden on us to show that the marketplace can do better rather than continuing to just say it?

The way out of this ethical dilemma is to have a single-payer system in which all are treated equally and health results become the standard for measurement. At present, the marketplace pays for process rather than outcome, and prevention is not a billable commodity. In the single-payer system, payments could highlight results in terms of morbidity and mortality. Results cannot always be measured for individual patients, but aggregate results can point out which programs should receive financial rewards.

This problem is not limited to medicine. The people for whom we vote make decisions on food stamps, medical coverage, education support, and research appropriations. When they vote not to provide early education, medical care, prevention, or Medicaid expansion, we as voters kill through errors of omission.

In addition, it is a false argument to say that it is either the marketplace or socialized medicine. Our military is superb. It is based on a single-payer system, but it is then expected to use the marketplace to acquire the commodities and systems required. Medical care could use the same approach. Somehow, the opponents of a single-payer system seem to imply that advocates are unpatriotic. The same argument is not made about advocating a single-payer system for the military.

And so public health must continuously be concerned with the harm resulting from actions taken, but especially it needs to be concerned with actions not taken. The dictum of First Do No Harm brings the ethical battlefield to budgetary medical ethics (2).

Ethical concerns are nothing new to public health.

Liquid Protein Diets

In 1976, *The Last Chance Diet* was published, and liquid protein diets became a popular way to lose weight (3). By August 1977, the FDA and the CDC had both received reports of women dying while using such a diet. In general, the reports were always of women, and they were usually young, in their thirties.

To provide context, what was happening in the other news at that time? A month earlier, the first oil flowed through the Alaska pipeline to Valdez. A week after the oil flow, President Carter created the Department of Energy. On August 16, Elvis Presley died at Graceland at age 42, and the Apple II computer went on sale. It was in the midst of this, that young women were dying as the result of a diet. EIS officers were dispatched. Together with the FDA, they studied more than thirty cases of sudden death. Since many of the deaths were in California, Rep. Henry Waxman (D-CA) held a hearing on December 28, 1977, in Los Angeles. He requested that I testify, together with the FDA, on the findings.

Semistarvation diets in previously obese persons warrant special attention to conduction problems of the heart. The consensus of those involved in this investigation was that somehow these deaths were indeed caused by cardiac conduction defects. The diets were quickly pulled from the market, but then a new and unexpected problem concerned the CDC. Senator Charles Percy, in his second term as a senator from Illinois, asked, through his staff, for the names of the women who had died. He wanted his Senate committee to conduct an investigation of the deaths to verify our results.

This was unprecedented for me, but I understood the logic of having an independent assessment. My concern was that the CDC investigators had provided assurances to the families that their information would be considered confidential. How could we furnish those names to a member of Congress?

My initial response to the Senate committee was to suggest that the CDC could provide the names to a separate nonpolitical medical group, such as the National Institutes of Health, for it to do an independent investigation. The Senate staff turned down this suggestion.

I then learned from the CDC legal counsel that I had no choice but to provide the names for two legal reasons. First, people lose their privacy at the time of death, so that privacy cannot be the reason for withholding names. Second, Congress has exempted itself from the Privacy Act; therefore, it can request and must receive information we would ordinarily consider private.

It was a disturbing position to be in. When I realized that I had no legal option, I called the Percy staff and asked whether they would be willing to issue a subpoena for the information. They said, "Of course." I had not expected them to immediately ask, "And then you will provide us with the names?" I said no, I would not, but we would then go to court, and the court would require that I give them the names. "If you already know the outcome," they asked, "why would you make the extra work for everyone?" I said it was because I wanted people to know that I had done my best to protect their privacy and that legally there was no more that I could do.

The interesting result was that they dropped their request rather than confront what might be adverse publicity for them. But this incident left me disturbed because the legal and ethical responses seemed to differ.

Hospital Infections

There were other dilemmas in the CDC's daily routines. Our laws are not always the best way to achieve health protection. On one occasion, an unusual organism was cultured from a person who had a new heart valve that had replaced a diseased valve. The hospital did the correct thing and called on the CDC to help trace the source of the infection. The unexpected finding was that this was not an infection caused by a break in the hospital's infection-prevention program. The infection was traced back to the valve manufacturer. In many ways, this is more serious because other hospitals would also be ordering valves from this supplier.

The case was reported in the *MMWR* to quickly alert the medical establishment. The hospital with the original infection was identified only as Hospital A in the report. After the report was published, a lawyer quickly filed a request for the hospital's name under the Freedom of Information Act. The lawyer then offered services to the patient, and they brought a $1 million lawsuit against the hospital. In a logical world, the hospital should not be held responsible for the contamination of the valve at the site where it was manufactured. Nonetheless, the hospital was faced with a lawsuit and, a model of cooperation to that point, it told the CDC it would never again report a hospital infection. The public did not win with that decision.

There are frequent calls for publication of infection rates by hospital, with the belief that patients are protected if they have this information and can then make the decision to avoid hospitals with high rates. Transparency should be the rule. But the public should also be warned that frequently the highest rates of reported infections are in hospitals with the best programs;

their rates are high because they have a functioning surveillance system. They actually seek and publish the results of their aggressive approach to reducing infections. Therefore, the risks may, in fact, be much higher in a hospital that reports a lower rate but has an inferior surveillance program.

Rates are also frequently higher in hospitals that care for many people who lack health insurance and who may enter the hospital in poorer physical condition than patients with good insurance coverage. A similar dilemma is seen in the reporting of hospital mortality rates; some of the best hospitals are faced with some of the most difficult cases. Such hospitals get these referrals because of their extensive experience and because they are often the hospital of last resort for some conditions.

Liquid protein diets and infected heart valves are the tip of the ethical dilemmas faced in public health. When we require immunizations for school entry, how do we compensate the small numbers who suffer adverse consequences from following the public health recommendations? In clinical medicine, reactions to penicillin or other drugs are accepted because those drugs are taken to treat an immediate threat, an infection. The risk-benefit discussion weighs taking the antibiotic versus the risk of not treating the infection.

The risks of Sabin polio vaccine were small but real. The risk of polio disease was even smaller but would increase if immunization rates fell. This difficulty finally led to a return to Salk inactivated vaccine in this country because it had no risk of disease associated with it. But the problem exists for other vaccines. What are the ethical obligations when we urge people to take the small risk of a vaccine side effect for the benefit of society?

What are the ethical implications of prescribing antibiotics for viral infections? Or of stopping a course of antibiotics when one feels better, even before the infection is adequately treated, thus giving the organism a chance to develop resistance? What are the implications of using antibiotics to speed the growth of animals, even if that also increases the risk of organisms' developing resistance?

Much of the increased life expectancy in the United States in the past century is due to prevention, vaccines, safer water supplies, food safety, reduced smoking rates, exercise, highway safety, sunblock, and millions of daily prevention decisions. How should we measure the harm caused when public health appropriations are inadequate?

chapter 17

GLOBAL HEALTH

Sharing Our Science

Global health interests were high at the CDC. The original tropical disease specialists influenced this atmosphere, and soon Robert Kaiser, an early EIS officer (class of 1959) and tropical disease expert, was in charge of a massive malaria program, funded by USAID. The program worked with a WHO plan to eradicate malaria. This program—in conjunction with the smallpox eradication activities, the posting of D. A. Henderson (also an EIS officer and epidemiologist) from the CDC to the WHO, and Alexander Langmuir's global interests—attracted globally inclined people to the EIS and other programs at the CDC.

However, the restrictions were significant. The CDC was expected to justify all global activities on the basis of improved health for Americans or as a response to a different funding agency, such as the USAID or the WHO. With these restrictions, Dave Sencer asked me to form a committee to advise him on how the CDC could best serve global health. Dave Sencer viewed health as one entire entity; he realized that what is good for the world is ultimately good for the United States. This perspective prompted him to detail many people to the Smallpox Eradication Program: he saw that the ultimate way to protect Americans from smallpox was to get rid of the disease everywhere. This strategy not only protected Americans but also was financially successful. The money that the United States contributed for smallpox eradication is recouped every three months. This is because adverse reactions to the vaccine that require hospitalization are absent, and approximately seven deaths a year, as the result of small-pox vaccine, are prevented. In the thirty-five years since smallpox was eradicated, the United States has seen its investment returned 140 times and avoided more than 225 deaths and literally thousands of vaccine complications.

This was the background for forming a group to advise Dr. Sencer on what the CDC could do to improve global health. The global health committee provided a specific recommendation. Because the CDC would probably never be a big funder for global health (this changed with AIDS and Ebola), the committee suggested that we identify the most important places in the world where global health decisions are made and then offer some of the CDC's best people on secondment to those places. The committee emphasized that assignments should go to people that the CDC valued and would want back. The committee concluded that the single most important decision-making place for global health was the WHO headquarters in Geneva, Switzerland. Further down the list were the WHO's regional offices, UNICEF, UNDP, and the World Bank. Sencer immediately began planning to offer a limited number of people the opportunity to work with the WHO in Geneva. The assignment of D. A. Henderson from the CDC to the WHO had already provided a precedent. Henderson headed up the WHO Smallpox Eradication Program for eleven years at WHO headquarters, always as an employee of the CDC. The ground rule with Henderson and those who followed was that the person would answer day to day to the WHO and not to the CDC. It was the only way of making the CDC employees a true gift to the WHO for the period that they were there, rather than a loan with conflicting loyalties.

The strategy worked. The WHO became even stronger when Rafe Henderson from the CDC was seconded to head up the Expanded Program on Immunization; Mike Merson, also a former EIS officer, was sent to direct the Diarrheal Disease Program and later the HIV/AIDS Program; and Jonathan Mann, another former EIS officer, was posted to work on AIDS. The WHO thus received strong management from people who could afford to do bold things. The CDC benefited by having staff acquire experience in global health decision making. The concept is still viable. Some WHO programs are funded outside its usual budget. Similarly, the WHO could have public health experts and managers assigned from various countries, who were not part of the WHO's personnel count, to augment its staff. The WHO must have the final word on agreeing to the assignee and the authority to terminate assignments not in its best interest.

When I became director, I wanted to continue to strengthen the global health contributions of the CDC. I felt that, for each disease or condition, a global view—rather than a domestic versus international view—was needed. Those working on respiratory viruses or enteric bacteria should see their field globally. For that reason, having the entire organization steeped in global health, rather than having a special program for global health, is best.

This commitment required specific attention to global aspects. The CDC had many international visitors for meetings and to take training courses. For many years, Ed Najjar did a superb job in facilitating international visitors' encounters with the CDC. Likewise, the CDC needed someone to coordinate all of its relationships with the WHO, UNICEF, the World Bank, and many other international agencies.

This led to our attempts to recruit Dr. Don Hopkins as deputy director for these global activities. Don was much sought after. He was a pediatrician who had global public health training under Dr. Tom Weller at Harvard. Harvard was offering Hopkins a position to stay with Weller's department. Hopkins had done an outstanding job on smallpox eradication while working in Sierra Leone and India; he was a self-starter, a good worker, and keen to improve global health. He was also being courted by Peter Bourne, who was working in the Carter administration.

We invited Don and his wife, Ernestine, to see the programs at the CDC. I had no idea that he disliked heights when we put him on one of the top floors at the Peachtree Plaza Hotel. Only years later did I discover that he had spent an anxious and often sleepless time during that visit. However, the potential at the CDC overcame the clumsy attempt at hospitality, and Don helped to put global health on the permanent agenda at the CDC.

The CDC global health story has many high and low points. A low point was the climate of racial unrest, which made housing difficult for scientists from other countries, particularly those from Africa. But this in turn led to a high point, in 1972, when the United Methodist Church, the Episcopal Church, the Evangelical Lutheran Church, the Presbyterian Church, the United Church of Christ, and the Atlanta Archdiocese Council of Catholic Women developed Villa International. Villa International is near the CDC and Emory University and offers short-term residence to persons of all faiths and from all parts of the world. It provides individual rooms but also a communal kitchen, which allows people to cook the foods they prefer. Since opening in 1972, Villa International has hosted more than 23,000 guests from 146 countries. While originally founded to host international guests of the CDC, the villa is open for scholars and researchers with short-term programs at other institutions, especially Emory.

Some events were particularly challenging. Soon after I became director of the smallpox program, David Sencer called me at home at dinnertime. He told me that the smallpox program would be accused of racism on the 10 p.m. news. His suggestion was that I go to the station and be prepared to appear on the news program to defend the program.

First, I had to know the issues. We were conducting a smallpox and global health–training program at the time, which included a dozen visitors from Nigeria. I was told that a local African American dentist had been in discussions with a number of the visitors, and he was charging discrimination. Specifically, he charged that their per diem rate was lower than that for Americans attending the training program and that the visitors were being housed in a roach-infested, second-class hotel.

There was no time to assemble all of the details before the news show, but I concluded that a white employee attempting to say that we were not involved in discrimination would look inappropriate. I called our new equal employment officer, Frank Miller, and begged for his help. Frank was an outstanding athlete (and a football teammate of Rev. Jesse Jackson in earlier years). Frank was new in this job, but he had a stellar reputation as a capable public health advisor with the Venereal Disease Program.

Frank agreed to appear on the program, and he provided a calm response and denied any discrimination. Years later, he told me that he did not know me at the time and was never sure why he had come to my rescue, but he did not regret it.

The event soon became even more painful when the CDC received a call from a viewer saying he intended to shoot the first African walking out the front door of that hotel. Once again, good people rose to the occasion. The Emory Inn, across the street from the CDC, called to say it would offer accommodations to the entire Nigerian delegation at the same prices as at the hotel in which visitors were then staying. Suddenly, the housing and the transportation concerns were solved.

It took some days to sort out the problem. In the end, it turned out that the Nigerian attendees were getting a *higher* per diem than the American attendees, not lower, because they were being paid by USAID, while Americans were subject to the rates provided by the CDC. Second, only three of the attendees were offended. They were physicians who were uncomfortable being treated the same as the nonphysician public health workers from Nigeria. These physicians pointed out that they would have received special treatment in their country or other countries, including limousines for the trip from the airport. One was especially offended that he had been picked up by a CDC smallpox employee in a pickup. Finally, it turned out that the delegation had been given the choice of accommodations and had selected that hotel in an attempt to save money, allowing them to return home with more gifts.

The local dentist received the publicity he sought, the three physicians seemed satisfied that they had made their point regarding their importance, and the remaining members of the delegation were deeply embarrassed and apologetic. I was subjected to questioning by the US Public Health Service (PHS) in Washington, DC, and was successfully defended by a senior PHS administrator, Paul Ehrlich, who later became the surgeon general. Figuring out the lessons learned in this incident was difficult. We could not treat the physicians differently from the rest of the delegation, but it pointed out the minefields when working with other cultures.

Despite such problems, dealing across cultures continued to be one of the true joys of working at the CDC. Over the years, we hosted visitors from dozens of countries, learned from their perspectives, and grew in our understanding of the world.

And often we shared humor. One visit of note included Dimitri Venediktov, deputy health minister in the Soviet Union. Venediktov was well known in global health circles, often representing the Soviet Union at international conferences. The *Bulletin of the World Health Organization* recounted, in October 2008 (1), his role in organizing the Primary Health Care conference in Alma Ata. This meeting established basic primary health care as a goal for all peoples of the world. David Tejada de Rivero, assistant director general of the WHO, related how Venediktov appeared at his home in January 1976 to say that the Soviet Union would provide $2 million to have a conference on primary health care in the Soviet Union. The previous May, delegates to the World Health Assembly had promoted such a meeting, but resources were not available.

Venediktov offered funding, the meeting was held, and it became a watershed moment in global health in promoting the idea of primary health care for all people in the world. It also resulted in tension between the WHO, which was promoting this concept, and UNICEF, which was promoting specific interventions under the name GOBI (for *g*rowth monitoring, *o*ral rehydration, *b*reastfeeding, and *i*mmunization). This tension interfered with basic health approaches because countries could not afford to offend either the WHO or UNICEF, and yet they were offering different visions on the road forward in global health. This tension continued until 1984, when the Task Force for Child Survival was formed, providing a common platform for immunization and then other programs of the two agencies.

Venediktov visited the CDC with his chief microbiologist, Viktor Mikhailovich Zhdanov. It was Zhdanov, who, as the deputy minister of health for the Soviet Union in 1958, called on the World Health Assembly to undertake an initiative to eliminate smallpox from the world. He left the Ministry of Health in 1961 to return to research. At the time of his visit to the CDC, his early efforts were being celebrated because smallpox had been eradicated.

Venediktov and Zhdanov were briefed by programs throughout the CDC and expressed their great respect for the work being done. But nothing intrigued them as much as the discovery of the *Legionella* bacterium. They both exclaimed that finding new human pathogenic viruses was expected, but to find a new human pathogenic bacterium took them completely by surprise.

On their final night at the CDC, we held a banquet at nearby Stone Mountain Park (site of the world's largest bas-relief carving), complete with Southern cooking. This was considered an important event by our government, and so Julius Richmond, the surgeon general, came in from Washington, DC, along with two State Department officials. Near the end of the dinner, I arose to offer the first toast. I suggested we toast the Soviet Army. The State Department officials blanched, the Soviet visitors suddenly appeared apprehensive, and only Dr. Richmond seemed relaxed.

I went on to explain that Bill Watson, deputy director of the CDC, had been a prisoner of war outside of Dresden in World War II. I explained the importance of Bill Watson for the health of Americans and indeed the health of people around the world. I then said it was his successful liberation by the Soviet Army that had made this all possible. The State Department officials began to breathe again, everyone cheered the Soviet Army, and the guests relaxed.

Dr. Venediktov then arose and said, "Americans bring out the competitive best in us. We have been greatly impressed with your accomplishments in isolating *Legionella*. We have agreed that we will now return home and attempt to find another human bacterial pathogen." He paused for a long moment before adding, "Even if we have to create it in the laboratory."

The success of the smallpox eradication effort improved the standing of the CDC. Requests continued to increase for consultation and for training of officers from other countries. Finally, the contribution that the CDC had sought to provide for years, namely, an expansion of both the CDC and the EIS to other countries, was achieved.

In 1976, Canada established the first Field Epidemiology Training Program (FETP) outside the United States, modeled after the EIS program at the CDC. In 1980, David Brandling-Bennett, a former EIS officer and tropical disease expert (later deputy director of the Pan American Health Organization, and even later an early scientist at the Bill & Melinda Gates Foundation), arrived in Thailand to initiate the first FETP outside of North America, at the request of the Government of Thailand. With initial funding from USAID, the program immediately demonstrated its value. Scientists in the program investigated infectious disease outbreaks, helped to characterize resistance patterns of antimalarial drugs, and became the gold standard for similar programs that developed in ensuing years in Asia. As in the United States, the program strengthened the entire public health infrastructure.

In the early 1980s, Secretary Richard Schweiker of the Department of Health and Human Services (HHS) attended the World Health Assembly. He asked me to send a paragraph to his speechwriter, offering US assistance in developing an EIS program for the WHO. Such assistance would have been an excellent way for the WHO to respond to health problems, train outbreak investigators from around the world, and strengthen its abilities to support such operations. A week later, Schweiker inquired about my paragraph. I said I had sent it. I re-sent it, but it still did not appear in his draft. The speechwriter did not want to include it. The secretary asked me to send it directly to him, and he included the offer in his talk. The offer was made to the WHO, but the organization did not accept it. Over the years, attempts were made to provide such a program. Rafe Henderson became an active promoter of the idea at the WHO. But the organization did not appreciate the potential of such a program, and the idea never achieved traction.

Despite the lack of enthusiasm at WHO headquarters, the concept spread to many countries. Such FETPs retained many attributes of the original EIS Program. The idea for all such programs is learning by doing. The number of persons trained each year is small, to allow for adequate supervision. In many programs, a laboratory component is part of the training so that epidemiology and bench science are combined. The CDC has now helped in developing over fifty such programs around the world. FETPs are country-owned programs, located within ministries of health, and are tailored to meet the public health needs of each country. They are a proud heritage of global health at the CDC.

The story isn't complete without mentioning that, for all of its proven worth of openness and transparency, the CDC approach of emphasizing global health is not automatic. Its value must be earned every day. The new century saw a different approach: the new HHS coordinator for global health under President George W. Bush issued an order that all WHO contacts must be centered in his office. If the WHO wanted a CDC expert on a committee, to provide consultation or to attend a meeting, the WHO was no longer free to go directly to the CDC, as had been done for decades. The WHO had to make the request through the Washington, DC, HHS office, and the coordinator would decide who attended the WHO meeting. It was a blow to improved global health. It is the kind of decision that controls a process rather than focusing on outcomes. There were, of course, consequences in terms of health. At times, the American attendee would be selected for political rather than for scientific expertise. The ability to provide informal consultation to WHO decisions was hampered, the CDC knowledge of what was happening globally was delayed rather than gathered in real time, and the WHO felt hampered in getting the best advice possible. However, in 2009, the CDC was once again able to provide direct leadership in global health.

People are often critical of the WHO—and for very good reasons. But if it didn't exist, it would have to be created. It operates with limitations that would not be tolerated by CEOs of other organizations. First, its "board of directors" consists of the ministers of health of all member countries. They meet annually, as the World Health Assembly, to decide on policies and programs and to review results. A board of 180 or 190 people is too unwieldy to be practical. In addition, ministers of health are generally political appointees, so they are not in office long enough to have a deep commitment to the WHO or to have an understanding of how to best support the organization for the benefit of the health of all people. Yet the practice has continued for more than sixty years. Practicality has ceased to be a consideration.

Second, at the formation of the WHO, the United States fought for it to have strong regional offices. This was done to protect the Pan American Health Organization, which had proved so effective in the Americas. It continues to be effective, but the WHO's other regions have become examples of what happens when politics becomes more important than health. Regional directors can be voted in one term after another by providing benefits to key people in key countries. Global headquarters in Geneva often lacks the resources or authority to implement needed global programs. In short, the world ties the hands of the director general.

Third, resources are inadequate for the task. The WHO operates a global organization on a smaller budget than that of the CDC. The WHO's annual budget for the entire world is about what diabetes costs the United States every week.

Fourth, in an attempt to represent the world, the personnel system tries to fill positions with an eye to balance. This isn't always the same as competence. For some employees, this is the best job they have ever had, and they cannot afford to jeopardize their employment with brave actions. Safe decisions become important.

After seventy years of experience, it is time to stop and ask what has been learned over that time and how we can revamp the WHO to be a more responsive and efficient program and a true leader in the improvement of global health. We are at a point where available tools, organizational ability, and interest make global health equity an achievable objective. How do we make the WHO as good as its potential? We could be doing much better.

Finally, it should be stressed that, while the CDC was already strong in global health for many years, it has now become truly global in its outreach. With literally hundreds of people assigned around the world, it is a major player in all WHO programs. But the CDC also responded with fieldworkers and major responsibilities when President George W. Bush launched the President's Emergency Plan for AIDS Relief (PEPFAR) with a commitment of $15 billion for five years (2003-2008). This program has had major success in treating AIDS patients throughout the world. It is a great and lasting legacy for President Bush.

chapter 18

POSITIVE POLITICS

Every public health decision also involves a political decision. Governments are the hope for public health and global health. Regardless of the high level of interest from church groups, NGOs, foundations, and service organizations, governments are the major funders of global health. While politicians may often be harmful to the health of people (as when they reduce support for immunization programs, refuse to expand Medicaid, or do not fund prevention in health care delivery programs), when properly motivated politicians can provide the strongest force in the world for positive change in health. Here is one example.

In early November 1979, Julius Richmond, surgeon general of the United States, called me to say that First Lady Rosalynn Carter was going to visit Cambodian refugee camps in Thailand, hoping to increase the world's response to the problems of the refugees. Illness and malnutrition were major problems, and the current response was not yet equal to the needs. Dr. Richmond had been asked to accompany Mrs. Carter. His concern was that he knew nothing about refugee camps. Because he knew I had worked in the Nigerian Civil War relief operation, he asked whether I would accompany him. I agreed.

We were briefed by various persons and groups, including former Assistant Secretary of Health Phil Lee. What impressed me was how definite the opinions were regarding the conditions, disease rates, and death rates, and yet the estimates varied widely; there seemed to be little factual evidence for those opinions. Many of the assertions seemed to contradict what the last briefing group had asserted. On something as straightforward as malaria rates or death rates in camp, there was no agreement.

We flew on what would have been Air Force One, if President Carter had been aboard, and made one stop for refueling in Anchorage, Alaska. On the flight, I was asked what malaria prophylaxis Mrs. Carter should take. I was on my own and could not seek the advice of the CDC's malaria experts. However, because of our time in Africa, I had followed the malaria prophylaxis and treatment literature to some degree. But now the saga of second-guessing began, and it ultimately led me to make the wrong decision—one that subsequently led to years of night sweats, as I would awaken to review my decision-making process on that trip. My first reaction, which was the correct reaction and the correct answer, was to say that we would be in an air-conditioned hotel in Bangkok for two nights and would be in the field only during the day, when mosquito bites are less frequent by malaria-transmitting mosquitoes. The risk of malaria would not be zero, but it would certainly be low. I had decided to take nothing myself, and I thought Mrs. Carter should not take any prophylaxis either. Then came the nagging doubts. What if the president's wife got malaria and the director of the CDC had been the one to advise her to skip prophylaxis? Malaria experts reading this will wonder why this was such a hard decision.

I went to the next step of my thinking, when I should have stopped thinking altogether. I had used chloroquine in Africa for both treatment and prophylaxis of malaria. But that drug had shown resistance in Thailand, and it made no sense to administer an ineffective drug. I had been told that embassy staff and others in Thailand were using a drug called Fansidar, a sulfa-based antimalarial. Given their experience, it seemed the best choice, but there was a downside. It had, at that moment, not yet been approved by the FDA. So what would be the implications of using a drug not licensed in the United States, if we encountered a problem? Dr. Richmond and I discussed it and decided that Fansidar was still the most prudent approach. We would wait and have the embassy in Thailand get the drug for Mrs. Carter. And that is what we did. Everything seemed to work fine.

Years later, the rest of the story appeared, and that is what left me waking up sweating in the middle of the night. The CDC issued the *MMWR* each Friday morning. It combined statistics on disease occurrence with articles on current public health problems. When I was director, the protocol included a block of time every Wednesday noon for me to do a final review of the *MMWR* before it was sent to press. This started my habit of reviewing the *MMWR* every week. Thus, in January 1985, I was reviewing the issue that had a lead story on deaths from Stevens-Johnson syndrome following the use of Fansidar! (This syndrome can result in devastating lesions and ulcers of the skin and mucous membranes. It can lead to pneumonia and organ failure and is a distressing complication.) The possibilities continued to haunt me for many years.

In Thailand, Dr. Richmond and Mrs. Carter made the rounds of camps. She had asked me before we left, what risks she would be taking by holding refugee children. Dr. Richmond was especially concerned about tuberculosis. My response was that the risk was small but not zero. While some children in camp undoubtedly had tuberculosis, they were not great transmitters, and I thought the upside of her showing her concern for the children in camps outweighed the theoretical risk of disease transmission. Her innate concern for the children—the concern that had brought her there in the first place—won out.

In the meantime, I was able to spend the day with two experienced CDC employees, Roger Glass, a former EIS officer, and Joe Giordano, former public health advisor and program manager of the Epidemiology Program at the CDC. Having arrived only days before we did, they had made incredible advance preparations for our visit.

It was clear in the crowded camps that there was no room to bury the dead. Roger and Joe found that there was a contract for the removal of bodies and that while there were not records by individual name, the contractors did get different compensation for children than for adults. Therefore, there was a numerator of deaths for every day for adults and children. Moreover, there was a count of people as they entered the camp. Thus, it was possible to construct death rates by day for each camp.

Glass and Giordano had also found a Walter Reed team investigating malaria so it was possible to get malaria rates and treatment outcomes.

The population pyramid was telling. There were children younger than age 6 months, fewer than expected between 6 and 12 months of age, and then almost no children from ages 1 to 6. Clearly, children who were breastfeeding had an advantage, but children ages 1 to 6 did not compete well for food and were therefore almost nonexistent.

On the plane during our return flight, I briefed Dr. Richmond on our findings. He was so impressed that we actually had numbers and graphs that he asked me to brief Mrs. Carter. I told her about the information gathered on the population pyramid, death rates by day, and disease rates. When I showed her the figures on deaths per day, I was able to put them in a broader context. Because of my review of the literature during the Nigerian

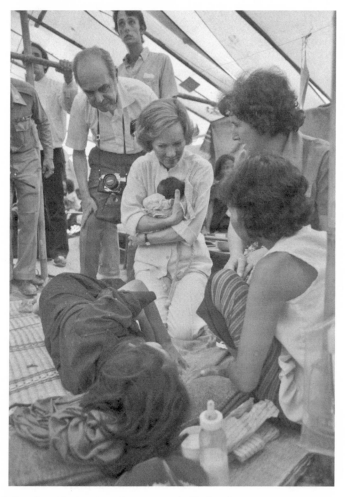

First Lady Rosalynn Carter at a refugee camp in Thailand. Photo from the author

Civil War, I had information on what was known about death rates in refugee camps and was able to compare the findings to other historical events. I told her that I knew of no situation worse than the Leningrad blockade, a 900-day siege of that Russian city during World War II. Vital statistics were kept, and as I recalled it, the Russians reached their worst level just before a relief road over the frozen lake allowed Soviet convoys to enter Leningrad in January 1942. At that point, bringing in some food and removing some of the people became possible. Death rates, as I recalled, were at about 1 per 1,000 per day, or 36 percent on an annual basis. In the refugee camps in Thailand, death rates were actually at the same level when the camps were first formed but rapidly declined as medical and nutritional programs responded to the needs. This comparison to Leningrad reinforced the seriousness of the refugee experience in Thailand but also reinforced the belief that quickly responding to these needs was possible.

Subsequently, a situation worse than Leningrad has occurred—the Rwanda genocide, where refugee camp death rates as high as 4 per 1,000 per day were recorded. At that rate, an entire camp would die in less than a year.

Several days after returning to the United States, the White House hosted a meeting, chaired by Father Theodore Hesburgh of Notre Dame, to hear a report from Mrs. Carter and to make recommendations on future actions. What happened next surprised me. The fact that Mrs. Carter was involved helped to mobilize efforts in both the United States and the world, and refugee aid increased in Thailand at an unbelievable speed. Once again I was reminded that every public health decision ultimately rests on a political decision.

Over time my interest in this relationship between politics and public health evolved. My early reaction was unhappiness with political decisions that hurt the public health through unnecessary suffering, early death, or compromised life quality. One day, my coworker Bill Watson took me to task, saying that the proper response to unwise political decisions should be to take responsibility. This led to the second step in my evolution. When politicians make bad decisions, he said, it is because they don't have the correct information at the right time, and I should take responsibility for that. (In general, this is true, but in recent years, it is disheartening to see adequate factual information on global warming and gun deaths be readily available but ignored by political decision makers. Mark Twain once said the person who doesn't read has no advantage over the person who can't read. Likewise, persons who do not use their intelligence have no advantage over those who lack intelligence.)

I took Bill Watson's advice to heart, and we began asking what information politicians needed and whether we were getting it to them. We redoubled our efforts, and, indeed, being proactive made a difference. But it is labor intensive to assemble and distribute information, and the turnover of politicians is so great that it is a continual education process.

The third step in my evolution was to urge public health workers to contemplate becoming politicians. It would be far more efficient, could only improve the debate, and would give me great comfort in my waning years to know that public health workers were in politics, making decisions on life quality.

How Public Health Should Be Funded

I am heartened by the political figures who made impressive contributions to public health. Senator Mark Hatfield, chairman of the Senate Appropriations Committee, was a consistent supporter of public health and global health. At my final appropriations hearing, Hatfield asked the subcommittee chair if he could conduct the hearing as a favor to me. One of his unexpected questions was how I would suggest public health should be funded. I wish I had anticipated that question.

My response was that the country could make several changes. First, for some public health programs, the financial benefits can be shown to exceed the financial costs. For example, benefit-cost analysis has demonstrated that every dollar invested in vaccine programs saves ten to twenty times that amount in the direct and indirect costs that would be incurred if the disease were not prevented. To not fund such programs means we not only continue to have the human suffering, but we also lose money in the process. That makes no logical sense on fiscal or humanitarian grounds. Therefore, my first recommendation would be that programs with proven positive benefit-cost ratios should become entitlements and no longer compete with other public health programs. To avoid battles between executive and congressional offices, my suggestion was that the responsibility of determining which programs are in that category should be left totally to Congress.

My second suggestion was that public health expenditures should be indexed to total health expenditures. Health care expenditures continue to increase over the years, whereas public health and prevention expenditures were declining as a percent of total health spending. I would be willing to accept whatever the ratio was at that point in time and fix that rate by indexing in the future.

These two changes would be rational and would provide long-term stability to public health efforts. But I would add a third suggestion. We have the audacity to advise other countries on health improvements, while having a totally dysfunctional and inefficient health care system in this country. As mentioned in an earlier chapter, two of the major barriers to improved health in the United States are (1) our inability to implement what we know in prevention and (2) the marketplace dominance of health care. Both problems are correctable.

The first problem is certainly made worse by inadequate public health resources, but it is also exacerbated by a system that penalizes attempts to deliver prevention in the health care system. Public health resources would be improved by my first two suggestions to the Senate subcommittee. But the inability of the health care delivery system to deliver prevention is criminal. Doctors are compensated for their interactions with a patient, usually to solve the complaint that brought them to the doctor. Physicians have guidelines on the average amount of time available for patients with various problems. But the system does not compensate physicians for time spent advising on tobacco use, exercise, diet, or safety measures. Therefore, practitioners cannot spend time on what they know would be useful to their patients and still make a living.

The marketplace is the other barrier, and it has failed the American public. Over a half-century ago, as I was completing my training, the American Medical Association bombarded us with materials on the King-Anderson bill, on how such efforts in political circles would reduce the freedom of doctors to make their own decisions and on the dangers of socialized medicine. Never did that organization point out that the marketplace might be more dangerous to the health of Americans than socialism would be. But that is exactly what has happened. When profit became the bottom line, quality, equity, and outcomes all suffered. Compensation began to focus on process, rather than on outcomes; the ease of measuring process, in terms of laboratory tests completed, CT scans performed, and the like, simplified paying for care. The great debates focused on quality, cost, and *access* rather than on quality, cost, and *outcomes*.

The marketplace is such a good mechanism for so many things that some assume it is a good mechanism for everything. Congressman Ron Paul once said that H1N1 flu is not something the government should respond to, that we should leave things this complicated to the marketplace. He made that remark only four years after the marketplace had demonstrated that it could not even manage the marketplace, much less influenza.

We simply cannot rely on the marketplace to reduce the health impact of tobacco when profits are made by selling tobacco. We cannot rely on the marketplace to reduce the risk of antibiotic-resistant bacteria. The great improvements in global health, in recent decades, are not the result of the marketplace. We should monitor the marketplace, and when it hurts the health of people, we need to find ways to correct the problem. Currently, the US marketplace has allowed the price of medical care to be higher per capita than any other country, and, despite that expenditure, we cannot even be in the top twenty countries of the world in terms of health outcomes. It is an absolute embarrassment for a country that prides itself on its can-do attitude and management skills.

Earlier I argued for a single-payer system. But is there a way to correct both barriers with one approach that uses the marketplace for delivery? Possibly. In 1993, the World Bank's annual report focused on health. It unveiled a new metric called disability-adjusted life years (DALYs), which for the first time provided a logical approach to combining suffering and death into a single number. Suddenly, a reasonable way to decide on priorities and to make decisions on resource allocation was made available.

Expecting to measure health outcomes for each individual patient is fraught with problems. The problems with DALYs are known, and it should be possible to develop improvements to measure health outcomes in the aggregate. The next improvements in DALYs could include a way to measure life quality. It could also fine-tune the problem of life value at different ages and refine the estimates of the suffering caused by various conditions. And the measure of suffering as a percentage of death requires much discussion. It would then be possible to allot a percentage of the payments to health plans on the basis of health outcomes for the aggregate, even though much of the payment would still be based on process measures. Beginning with 5 percent or 10 percent of total payments on this basis could provide the incentive needed for health programs to focus on outcomes in addition to process.

A financial return to plans with better health outcomes would lead to incorporation of programs on smoking cessation, nutrition, exercise, and state-of-the-art education on diabetes and hypertension, to name a few. In short, there would be a reason to incorporate prevention practices into health care delivery because it would be profitable.

Success with this approach would allow other experimentation. For example, special financial incentives could be provided for improved health outcomes of defined special high-risk groups. These could include people who are overweight and those who have diabetes or hypertension, for example. This approach could provide financial incentives for enrolling the sickest people rather than the healthiest.

In this case, the marketplace could respond to specific targets, and it might be possible to demonstrate that we could again provide leadership to the world by improving health at a reasonable cost. It will require obsessive attention to prevention and the constant question, why prevention? To save money? . . . Yes, but it is far more than that. It is simply better to be well than sick, alive than dead, and healthy than disabled. The reason for prevention is to improve the quality of life.

chapter 19

TOXIC POLITICS

Politicians were responsible for some of the most difficult problems we faced. Not all bullies end up in politics. But some do, and they find the rules favor the bully. The system is definitely stacked in favor of politicians and against workers in government programs. Testifying at a congressional hearing makes this clear. The room is set up to illuminate one part of the caste system in our society. Congressmen and senators sit on an elevated platform, always looking down on the witnesses. In a courtroom, having the judge elevated may be appropriate, but the practice seems like overkill in Congress—or at least an effort at false importance.

Some members of Congress would attempt to establish a sympathetic environment to let you know they were interested in the hearing or the problem at hand. But many established from the beginning that you were an enemy, as a government employee, and they, the politicians, had the most power.

Philip Zimbardo's famous experiment at Stanford University demonstrated how quickly students who were assigned randomly to be guards or prisoners began to alter their behavior to actually live those roles. The power of being a guard caused good people to become abusive. Zimbardo's book (1) applies the lessons learned in that classroom experiment to actual life situations with prison guards or with priests preying on children. He points out that these aren't problems of "bad apples" but rather of "bad barrels," in which the social situation alters the behavior of good people.

Not all politicians act out the power they have been given in unacceptable ways. Senators Dale Bumpers, Paul Simon, Mark Hatfield, Ted Kennedy, Bob Graham, Bill Lehman, and Richard Schweiker and Congressmen Paul Rogers and Henry Waxman never seemed to abuse their power. They demonstrated that it was possible to exercise the political role humanely and successfully.

One of the most extraordinary examples of genuine kindness happened one day when I was to testify in front of Senator Schweiker. A contentious problem was being discussed, and the room was filled, with standing-room only. As I stood in back waiting for a panel to finish testifying before I took my turn at the witness table, Senator Schweiker spotted me, sent an aide to ask me to follow him, and took me to sit next to him as the panel was questioned. It was uncomfortable for me, as the panel could see I was getting special attention and would soon counter their testimony, but it filled me with respect for the senator.

I watched my predecessor, David Sencer, absorb egregious political criticism over the Swine Flu Vaccination Program, as well as over the investigation of Legionnaires' disease (see chapter 9). Congressman John Murphy of the 17th District of New York was unceasing in his criticism.

One congressman from the South, Congressman William Natcher, a fine and fair person at hearings in most regards, would start each appropriations hearing by asking me whether I knew Dr. Ted Cooper. I would answer that I did and that he oversaw the CDC in my earlier years, as the assistant secretary of health.

"Do you respect Dr. Cooper?" he would ask. I would say that I did.

"Is he recognized as being a good scientist?"

Yes he is, I would respond. He would then read a quote from Dr. Cooper taken many years earlier to the effect that he did not think smoking was a significant health problem. Having made his point for his tobacco-growing constituents, Natcher would then proceed with the appropriations hearing.

Some politicians seemed fair in many respects but were willing to make decisions against the health of people for their own personal gain. People who take a daily vitamin pill with breakfast assume it is safe and approved by the FDA. However, because of Senator Orrin Hatch, the FDA lost its ability to control vitamins and supplements with passage of the Dietary Supplement Health and Education Act of 1994. These products have no federal scientific oversight and are not required to use truth in advertising. A number of the nutritional supplement programs are based in Utah, Hatch's home state, and in 2003, it was reported that Hatch owned shares in at least one nutritional supplement company. But Hatch was simply a leader. A majority had to vote *with* him to make this happen. It is a sad commentary on our elected officials and the influence they have on our lives.

My own theory is that we were fortunate to have such enlightened founding fathers. How could we have expected to get Washington, Jefferson, Adams, Franklin, and their ilk from such a small population base? And why do we not see that quality in politicians today? Perhaps because in the late eighteenth century, outlets for people with intellectual gifts were limited. They could go into teaching, theology, or politics. Now the opportunities are boundless for the curious and gifted. They can go into multiple fields of science, computing, teaching, theology, and business, to name a few. We are left with a diminished percentage of the gifted who find their passion in politics, and this may well be skewed toward those seeking attention who are also able to get financial backing. In that sense, as Lincoln Steffens asserted a century ago, *representative* government may be difficult to achieve.

Some politicians were more difficult to figure out. Congressman Ted Weiss represented much of Manhattan's West Side and was very popular. Indeed, a federal office building on Broadway was named in his honor. His story is a typical American immigrant success story. His family fled the Nazis in 1938 for the United States. He grew up in New Jersey and received a law degree from Syracuse University. He became a naturalized citizen, worked for the district attorney in New York, and then entered politics. He was a strong supporter of civil rights. Nothing in his history would have predicted the problems he caused us.

Congressman Weiss asked to inspect our files on human immunodeficiency virus (HIV) and AIDS. Since he represented a district with many cases, it was natural that he would be interested in the problem. I informed him that we would accommodate his request, but it would take us some time to remove all identifiers, such as the actual names of AIDS patients. He then held a press conference to say that he suspected the CDC had information on AIDS that we were not sharing with him or the public. He asked whether he could send an assistant to the CDC to review our files on AIDS. I said he could but repeated that we would remove identifying information on the names of patients, and that we would do this for privacy reasons.

The investigator came and said that the congressman wanted the full files, including the names of patients. We stood firm and refused to release patients' names. To my surprise, I received a letter from the congressman attempting to bully me into acquiescence; the letter stated that he was interested in the entire file, including the names of patients.

My refusal led him to another press conference, in which Weiss talked about my refusal to let Congress see the records, never mentioning that the contentious issue was his request for the names of AIDS patients. He simply said that he had asked for the whole file, and I insisted on redacting the files before sharing them. He then said he would call for a hearing at which I would be questioned. I decided on my approach but did not share what I planned to do with my superiors. At the hearing, I was accompanied by my supervisor, Ed Brandt, assistant secretary for health and a scientist of the highest ethical standards. The congressman started by castigating me and my lack of cooperation with Congress. He painted me in unflattering terms and then asked me for my statement.

I thanked him and then held up his letter to me and asked for his permission to include this letter (asking for the personal identifiers of people with AIDS) into the record of the hearing. Because other committee members were present, he could not refuse my request. The letter exposed his duplicity of asking for information on the names of persons with AIDS, while publicly denying that he had made such a request. This changed the tenor of the hearing.

Congressman Obey

Perhaps the most difficult of all congresspeople for me to deal with was David Obey from Wisconsin's 7th District. With so many good qualities and his genuine interest in education, health, and the environment, he was nonetheless a bully.

I intended to put one of the CDC's best scientists into a particular position when I received a call from Congressman Obey's office to say that the scientist's nomination would be a mistake. I did not know at the time that the scientist in question had once investigated an outbreak in Obey's district and had given a statement to a reporter on his interpretation of the problem. The scientist was unaware that his interpretation was counter to what Congressman Obey had told the press. The congressman was not pleased.

I was next surprised to get word from Secretary Califano's office requesting that I withdraw the scientist's nomination. My concern was that the administration should not allow congressional influence on personnel decisions within agencies. Congress has a quite different responsibility for high-level positions in departments. I did not heed the request and was told again, by an assistant to Secretary Califano, to withdraw the nomination.

When I again refused, the secretary asked to see me. I never feared being fired. Because I always knew I could return to the field of global health, I could separate scientific decisions from personal ramifications. Nonetheless, it is anxiety-producing to know you are about to be reprimanded. I entered his office, knowing it would not be pleasant but also believing that a principle was involved. The secretary had just completed a run and was in sweat clothes with his feet propped up on the desk.

He said, "I have asked my staff to ask you to withdraw the nomination, and there has been no action. What is the problem?" Recall that I had not sought this job. I was enjoying it but would enjoy other things also. So I replied, "The problem is that I know the difference between right and wrong, and your staff is trying to get me to do wrong." His feet immediately hit the floor; he sat up and said, "Let's hear your side of the story." Secretary Califano was a demanding boss in many ways because he expected everyone to work as hard as he did. But he was a good boss. You could expect his full support on projects of importance, and he showed himself to be, above all, fair.

When I finished, he said he understood and would not force me to do that. But he said that he had a friendly relationship with Obey and therefore could not help me. I would be on my own. I said I understood . . . but perhaps I didn't.

Sometime later, I received a call directly from Congressman Obey. He was angry. He was not calling me to discuss the situation. He was calling me with a naked threat. He said, "I will get you, and I will get the CDC. If you think I can't do that, wait until you come up for your next appropriations hearing."

The hearing was everything Obey said it would be. The CDC hearing was supposed to be two hours long, followed by an appropriations hearing for the Health Services Administration. When I realized how hard it was going to be, I decided to simply bear it but to avoid letting Obey see me get rattled or angry. So I just answered his questions, as inane as they became.

"How much does the CDC spend on printing each year?"

My response was, "I don't know the figure but will get it and provide it for the record."

"You mean you are the director of the CDC and you don't know how much you spend on printing?"

"That's right, but I can get the information for the record."

And so it went, question after ridiculous question, for the next four hours. He called a break for lunch and said we would continue after lunch.

Meanwhile, Dr. George Lythcott, director of the Health Services Administration and the former chief of the CDC Regional Office in Lagos, Nigeria, had appeared for his hearing, sat through two hours of my hearing, and could not figure out what was going on. At the break for lunch, George asked me, "What in the world is happening?"

I reassured him that Congressman Obey would be docile by the time George testified. I told George, with much sarcasm, "I think I have him on the run." Indeed, I did. You cannot continue to ask such questions without your colleagues on the committee beginning to wonder about your motives. But it always made me wonder whether he knew how much trouble he was causing.

Next, I heard from an influential health leader that Congressman Obey had informed him that I was the single biggest threat to disease prevention in the United States. We have some major threats, such as tobacco, but now I was being classified as even worse than tobacco.

Politics and NIOSH

But this bizarre story was not yet complete. The National Institute for Occupational Safety and Health (NIOSH) was a division of the CDC. It was the most political program in the CDC at that time because workers were interested in safer working conditions and corporations were interested in profit. It often came down to management versus labor, and both groups would lobby Congress. Congress therefore had an interest in this program that it might not have in most CDC programs.

The program headquarters were located in Washington, DC. And while NIOSH included fine scientists with many working in other locations, it was subjected to political forces that often made it difficult to use the science fairly.

I became convinced that NIOSH headquarters should be moved out of Washington for a number of reasons. The first was to get the headquarter's staff away from the political pressures that seemed inherent in that location. A second reason was to provide synergy with the Center for Environmental Health. The issues for the two programs were similar, except that one had to do with the time on the job and the other with the time off the job. Both dealt with injuries and chemical exposures, for example. It was my hope that in the future the two programs would actually be merged. It made scientific sense to avoid duplication of effort. That could not happen until NIOSH became less political and the Center for Environmental Health became stronger and more robust.

Dr. Julius Richmond, the assistant secretary for health, was sympathetic but could not see a way to do it. When Ed Brandt became assistant secretary for health in the Reagan administration, he reexamined the issue and became strongly convinced that NIOSH should be housed in an area of science rather than in an environment of politics.

The NIOSH staff was strongly resistant to the idea of moving their headquarters to Atlanta. Another scenario was developing at this time. It involved an attempt by some politicians and some NIOSH staff to move the institute to NIH. Since NIH headquarters were already in the Washington area, if NIOSH answered to NIH, attempts to move NIOSH headquarters to Atlanta would be halted.

Several leadership changes at NIOSH complicated the issue. Director Jack Finkle resigned in March 1978. J. Donald Millar was acting director for a year until Tony Robbins took the position in 1979. After Robbins left, Millar became the permanent director in 1981. He provided solid, long-term leadership to NIOSH and made it a better organization.

Before Millar became director, the attempted move to NIH became serious. We learned that NIOSH staff members were working with Congressman John Dingell, who had agreed to take the lead to get NIOSH moved to NIH. We also learned that Dingell planned to bring it up as an incidental floor motion; this move would take people by surprise and would minimize opposition. The decision would be made before we would know the issue was going to be raised. We pretended to know nothing about these efforts, but Bill Watson, deputy director of the CDC, along with George Hardy, the CDC's representative in Washington, lined up people who were willing to resist such a move. The problem was that we would have to know when the motion was coming to the floor to be sure those people were actually in the chambers. We were not quite sure how to determine that.

And then fortune blessed us. I was chairing a session in Texas at the American Public Health Association annual meeting. The session was the first item on the program that morning. Tony Robbins was supposed to be on the panel, but when I got there a few minutes early, I learned that Tony had been called back to Washington the night before. I went to a pay phone, called Bill Watson, and we guessed that this was the day for the floor motion. I returned to the panel in Texas, while Bill Watson put our plan into action.

We were correct. Dingell made the motion on the floor with some disparaging remarks about the CDC's stewardship of the program. He then proposed righting this wrong by moving NIOSH to be supervised by NIH. But then, seemingly out of nowhere, various people surprised Dingell with forceful statements opposing the motion, and it went down in defeat. I had a chance to watch the proceedings later on CSPAN. The plotters had no idea why that plan was killed.

With the help of Ed Brandt, we began planning to move NIOSH headquarters to Atlanta. Those in Congress who wanted continual political input into occupational health issues were not about to let that happen.

Congressman Obey effectively killed the plan when he put a rider on the CDC appropriations bill specifically prohibiting the use of money to move NIOSH. He knew how to play the game, and we were neophytes. We appeared stymied.

I became acquainted with Senator Mark Hatfield of Oregon when he called me to his office to ask questions about the health problems of Africa. We continued to discuss a number of issues, and I regarded him as a wise and sensitive person. I asked his advice on the NIOSH move. When I explained the problem, he immediately agreed it was the right thing to do but said it would be very difficult to get around a savvy person like David Obey. But he said if we had our minds made up that this was the correct thing to do to improve health, and if we could have all the plans made to actually make the move, there would be a day when the CDC might have a continuing resolution regarding their appropriations. That would, for a short period of time, not include the restrictions inserted by Congressman Obey. If we could move fast during that window, it would be legal to do so, but of course we would have to be prepared for the political fallout of an angry Obey.

Sometime after this advice was given, a representative from Obey's office, a public health professional, came to see us at the CDC. Clearly, he had been sent by Obey, but he presented himself as a public health professional wanting to help the CDC. He said he was well aware of the problems we had with Obey and that Obey had with us. He wanted us to understand that Obey was a power player. He knew how to use power and was unafraid to do so. "Someday," he said, "he will be the chair of the Appropriations Subcommittee and then the full committee." (This became true in 2006.) The representative for Obey went on to say that the "CDC's budget at that time would be totally dependent on him." He said that Obey was angry with me, but if I would make a public statement saying I was wrong and that I had decided against moving NIOSH, he thought Obey would reward the CDC with more resources.

During this discussion, Carol Walters brought me a note to say that Senator Hatfield was on the phone. I excused myself to take the call. Senator Hatfield told me that there would be a continuing resolution before the end of the week. This was our chance, but we didn't know whether the continuing resolution would last for days or for weeks. I told Bill Watson, who got the process started to move NIOSH headquarters from Washington, DC, to Atlanta on the following Saturday.

I went back to the meeting and was much more congenial. I told the person how pleased I was that he took the time to give us his ideas and suggest some options. Now we would have to discuss the ideas and make some decisions. In my mind, I watched him going to the airport, calling Obey to say he thought he had convinced us.

NIOSH was moved that weekend, Obey fumed, and NIOSH became a better program as it entered a scientific environment and the opportunity to work with environmental health staff over the next years. As director, Don Millar brought no-nonsense science to the enterprise. I saw that a merging with environmental health was a possibility in the future to the benefit of public health.

But the future is hidden from us. Bill Clinton became president; he named Dr. Phil Lee as the assistant secretary for health (his second time in that position) and—after pressures in Washington, DC, that I don't understand— Lee made the decision to move NIOSH headquarters back to Washington. I wrote Lee a memo on why a move back to Washington would once again compromise the health of Americans. He sent the memo to David Satcher, the new director of the CDC, with a personal note, asking Satcher to fix my unhappiness. It is not helpful for new directors to be plagued by old directors, so having expressed my concerns, I withdrew from the fight. Our hard-won victory was undone in a moment by politics, and David Obey won in the end. But public health did not win.

chapter 20

REYE SYNDROME

Following the Evidence

Sometimes a disease problem descends abruptly, as with the first case of Lassa fever in the United States in 1969. Sometimes the problem is abrupt but the explanation delayed, as with Legionnaires' disease in 1976. But often the problem is understood only over time, when enough evidence is finally available to allow for insights.

This chapter highlights the agonizingly slow unraveling of a problem and the equally slow steps in responding adequately to it. Part of the problem was working in a field at the edge of the science. At the time of this outbreak, we in the public health world did not even know how to do meta-analysis (a mathematical approach of putting studies together to give the aggregate findings more power than the individual observations), and, therefore, we could not assemble experiences into a convincing whole. One enemy was a powerful aspirin industry, which did not want to lose profits from giving aspirin to children, even if it could be harmful.

This account appears repetitious at times but that only points out the careful line we had to walk in uncovering the truth. This account may also read more like a scientific report than a story of solving a mystery, but that is also the point. It shows science at its best, finally leading to a policy change and then a behavioral change.

Reye syndrome, or Reye's syndrome, took time to understand. The condition may have been recognized in the 1920s. However, it was a paper by Reye,

Morgan, and Baral, in the *Lancet* in 1963 (1), that gave it the status of a syndrome, and suddenly many pediatricians realized that they might have seen the condition. This syndrome is characterized by fever, lethargy, confusion, and vomiting and may include a rash on the hands and the feet. The injury is most pronounced in the brain and the liver. Adults are rarely affected. Children may go into coma or have seizures; children die in one-third of cases.

Shortly after the *Lancet* paper, EIS officer George Johnson reported on an outbreak affecting sixteen children with influenza B who developed neurologic symptoms and signs (2). It was the beginning of a frustrating journey to investigate a mystery while fighting off snipers from industry and government.

Arizona Study

In 1979, Karen Starko, another EIS officer, conducted a study in Phoenix, Arizona, that finally provided traction for public health action. She reported, along with her colleagues, on seven pediatric cases of Reye syndrome during an influenza A outbreak. These scientists compared the course of these children's illness and treatment with those for sixteen control classmates who had also been sick but had not developed Reye syndrome (3).

All the patients had taken medications for their influenza symptoms. Whereas all seven case-patients had been given salicylates (that is, nonsteroidal anti-inflammatory drugs such as aspirin), only half of the sixteen controls had received these drugs. While the numbers were small, this was a turning point in understanding the risk of aspirin for this condition.

A July 1980 *MMWR* review (4) reported on more than 300 cases of Reye syndrome in a four-month period. It spoke of the association of the syndrome with certain viruses and other "factors, such as medications or toxins" that might contribute to the disease. Among the toxins were "isopropyl alcohol . . . warfarin, and aflatoxins." It then mentioned the Starko study before concluding that "further investigations are needed to more clearly define the possible role of salicylates use and toxins in the pathogenesis of Reye Syndrome."

Ohio and Michigan

On November 7, 1980, the *MMWR* reported on studies in Ohio and Michigan that added to the 7 cases reported by Starko. Michigan reported on 25 patients, and Ohio collected 159 cases from pediatric centers. These studies included control groups. The editorial comment stated: "The results of these studies suggest that during certain viral illnesses the use of salicylates—even before the onset of vomiting—may be a factor in the pathogenesis of Reye syndrome. *In view of these data, parents should be advised to use caution when administering salicylates to treat children with viral illnesses, particularly chickenpox and influenza-like illnesses* [emphasis added]" (5).

Looking back, the reader may be bewildered by the CDC's reluctance to provide stronger warnings. The problem was a desire to show "statistical significance" before making a recommendation.

The following month, in December 1980, Starko and her colleagues published the results of their 1979 study in the journal *Pediatrics* (3). Now their findings were in a peer-reviewed journal, not just a government publication. As the evidence mounted, there were great efforts to test the validity of these findings. While control groups increase confidence in findings, it is always possible that parents' recall is different because their children were severely ill, whereas the control children were less so. It is also possible that the more severe illness of Reye syndrome led to the increased use of aspirin rather than the other way around. And could the investigators have "led the witness" by a preconceived idea that aspirin was a hazard? For all of these reasons, some suggested using caution about recommending against the use of aspirin in these cases.

February 1982 CDC Statement

By late 1981, the CDC concluded the evidence was sufficiently strong that "caution when administering salicylates" was no longer sufficient. The association was strong, but causality was more difficult to prove. After consulting various groups, we decided to be totally transparent in saying that causality could not be proved but that doctors and parents were entitled to have all of the information that we possessed. Plans were made to publish the accumulated information plus the recommendation to withhold aspirin from children having chickenpox or flu in the *MMWR* on February 12, 1982.

The pressure from aspirin manufacturers took me by surprise. One would think that if a problem existed with aspirin use in children with influenza or chickenpox, the manufacturers would want to know that to protect both children and themselves. That was not the reaction at all. First, representatives from the aspirin manufacturers came to the CDC with boxes of "new" data, which we were obliged to examine. We found nothing new, but it took weeks of study to determine that. Next, the aspirin manufacturers began sending me messages, calling me at home and even at my parents' home when I went for a visit. The messages and pleas were varied, but the bottom line was always that the CDC's reputation was at stake and did I want to be the one that ruined its record for scientific integrity? All it would take is to make an announcement that aspirin should not be given under certain conditions and if that proved to be incorrect, the CDC's reputation would be soiled. Then they would ask, "Do any of the studies reach statistical significance?"

We proceeded with plans to publish a review in the *MMWR*. The issue would also contain a joint statement with the FDA, issuing a stronger warning about the use of aspirin.

The night before publication of the *MMWR* article, I received a call from the FDA. That agency said that the aspirin manufacturers had come late that day with new information on the use of aspirin and Reye syndrome. FDA felt obligated to review that information and so could not sign on to a statement until that had been completed.

The aspirin manufacturers anticipated that the government would have to delay publication of a recommendation, and they may have gone to bed that night content that they had bought more time. Such stalling tactics could have continued on for an extended period. But the CDC took them by surprise. The next day, February 12, 1982, the *MMWR* article (6) was published without the FDA's signoff.

The *MMWR* reviewed what had happened since the original Arizona report on seven cases and indicated that a fourth study had now been reported. Michigan had conducted a second study during the 1979-1980 influenza season, concentrating on all medications used with attempts to get dosage figures and frequency of administration; this study had one to three controls for each patient. Interviews were conducted within days of the report of the case to improve the accuracy of reporting. All twelve case-patients had used salicylates versus 41 percent of the twenty-nine control children (6).

The CDC then went on to note, "After reviewing the data from all four studies and discussing the various epidemiologic and analytic methods and results, the CDC consultants concluded that it was unlikely for the limitations of the studies, either singly or in combination, to explain totally the strength and consistency of the observed association between Reye syndrome and salicylates." The consultants felt that there was "sufficient evidence to support the cautionary statements on salicylate usage that had been published previously by the Centers for Disease Control." Furthermore, it was the consensus of the consultants that "until the nature of the association between salicylates and Reye syndrome is clarified, the use of salicylates should be avoided, when possible, for children with varicella infection and during presumed influenza outbreaks." The report continued: "In summary, these studies indicate to CDC that salicylates may be a factor in the pathogenesis of Reye syndrome, although the observed epidemiologic association does not prove causality. The exact pathogenesis of this disease and the possible role of salicylates in its pathogenesis remain to be determined. Additional well-controlled studies are also needed. Until definitive information is available, CDC advises physicians and parents of the possible increased risk of Reye syndrome associated with the use of salicylates for children with chickenpox or influenza-like illness" (6).

It may not seem so, but this was a clear step beyond saying to exercise caution. It was a recommendation to withhold salicylates. The reaction was swift. The aspirin manufacturers went to my supervisor, Dr. Ed Brandt, assistant secretary for health at HHS. He could have referred them to me, saying he had not been involved in the statement. Instead, he told them that he fully supported my authority to publish the article and that he agreed with the conclusions.

The aspirin manufacturers then went to the secretary of HHS, Richard Schweiker, who also gave the CDC his full support. The manufacturers next went to the White House. And the White House ordered the CDC to "cease and desist" and to start a new study of the association of Reye syndrome and aspirin. This was done. But "cease and desist" orders from the White House were of little interest to pediatricians, and the order from the White House could not take away the words of that publication. Pediatricians stopped using aspirin during flu outbreaks and for chickenpox treatment.

Four months later, a Surgeon General Advisory was issued in the June 11, 1982, *MMWR* (7). This, of course, was an official statement and therefore cleared by the White House. The report said, "The Surgeon General notes that the matter has been reviewed recently by several groups from within and outside government" and went on:

• CDC, on the basis of its review of the available data and the recommendations of an advisory panel on February 12, 1982, stated that "until definitive information is available, CDC advises physicians and parents of the possible increased risk of Reye syndrome associated with the use of salicylates for children with chickenpox and influenza-like illness [6]."

• The American Academy of Pediatrics Committee on Infectious Diseases also has reviewed the data, and in the June 1982 issue of *Pediatrics* issued a statement advising that the use of salicylates should be avoided for children suffering from influenza or chickenpox. (8)

• A Food and Drug Administration (FDA) working group audited the raw data in February 1982 from 3 studies conducted by state health departments (2 in Michigan and 1 in Ohio) and independently analyzed the data. The FDA evaluation was discussed in an open public meeting sponsored by FDA, CDC, and the National Institutes of Health on May 24, 1982. Invited experts from the academic community, the drug industry, and consumer organizations attended the meeting. It was the consensus of the scientific working group at the completion of the meeting that the new analysis supported the earlier evidence of an association between salicylates and Reye syndrome. As a result of this entire review process, the Surgeon General advises against the use of salicylates and salicylate-containing medications for children with influenza and chickenpox.*

On January 11, 1985, the *MMWR* reported that "during 1982–1984, the annual incidence of RS [Reye syndrome] was the lowest reported since the initiation of national surveillance" (9). The report went on to describe the new study ordered by the White House:

A pilot study was conducted between February and March 1984 to determine the study feasibility and establish methodology. The pilot study included 29 RS cases and 143 controls consisting of children admitted to the same hospital (IP) or emergency room (ER), attending the same school, or identified by random-digit dialing (RDD). Ninety-seven percent of case children were reported to have received salicylates during the respiratory or chickenpox illness before a clini-

*The surgeon general used no reference but noted that the FDA would notify health professionals through its *Drug Bulletin* and would take the steps necessary to establish new labeling requirements for drugs containing salicylates.

cally defined onset of RS, compared with 28% (ER), 23% (IP), 59% (school), and 55% (RDD) at any time during their matched illnesses. The risk defined in the pilot study was comparable to or greater than that determined in the previous studies. The Institute of Medicine (IOM), National Academy of Sciences, served to advise and critique the protocol, monitor the study progress, and review study analysis and results.

The *MMWR* went on to state that, after the IOM reviewed the methods of data collection, in July 1984, and the data analysis, in December 1984, the IOM stated, on January 8:

1. The PHS Task Force should proceed with the full study.
2. Results of the pilot study should be released promptly to the public and to scientists for review and analysis.
3. Analysis of the pilot study data reveals a strong association between Reye syndrome and the use of aspirin; considering data from previous studies also show an association of use of aspirin and Reye syndrome, the Committee recommends that steps should be taken to protect the public health before the full study is completed.
4. Although it is impossible to know with certainty whether the release of the pilot study data will harm the full study, the Committee suspects the effects of the attendant publicity will be no more damaging than the current climate of public opinion, which appears not to have impeded conduct of the pilot study. (9)

The *MMWR* article concluded with the following: "A report of the pilot study is currently being prepared for publication. In view of these preliminary findings, physicians, parents, and older children who self-medicate should continue to be advised of the probable increased risk of RS associated with the use of salicylates for children, including teenagers, with influenza-like illness or chickenpox [reported by the Division of Viral Diseases, Center for Infectious Diseases, CDC; the Reye Syndrome Task Force, consisting of members from the FDA, NIH, and the Office of the Assistant Secretary of Health, and the CDC]" (9).

The Impact on Reye Syndrome

On February 7, 1986, the *MMWR* reported on the full 1985 Reye syndrome experience (10):

Following the results of the pilot phase of the U.S. Public Health Service study on RS and medications, the U.S. Food and Drug Administration has proposed that oral over-the-counter medicine containing aspirin add a label reading: WARN-ING: Children and teenagers should not use this medicine for chickenpox or flu symptoms before a doctor is consulted about Reye syndrome, a rare but serious disease.

For the 1985 surveillance year, 91 cases of Reye syndrome (RS) meeting CDC's case definition were reported. Although delayed reports through June 1986 may increase the number of cases for 1985, the provisional 1985 total is *less than half the lowest annual total* [emphasis added] reported through the National Reye Syndrome Surveillance System (NRSSS) since its initiation in December 1973.

In previous years, the RS incidence, at least in part, has reflected the intensity and type of influenza activity. By all surveillance parameters, 1985 influenza activity was comparable in intensity to 1984, and the activity was greater than in 1982 or 1983.

And so we saw the beginning of a solution to the Reye syndrome problem. It involved all of the fears of parents; the suffering of children; the mystery of causation; the use of surveillance systems; epidemiology, risk calculations, and understanding the implications of government statements; the clash of the marketplace and public health; both the beneficial and problematic roles of government; and, finally, a solution communicated to medical workers and the general public to alter behaviors. The foundations of the solution were science and a systematic reduction of uncertainty until the association of aspirin in causing this problem could not be ignored. The system worked once again but not before many had their patience tested and many others suffered an unnecessary illness or death.

chapter 21

COMIC RELIEF

The work at the CDC is important, serious, and often intense. Our global health work often occurred against a dark background of suffering, death, and impaired quality of life.

Saving one child from measles is not much of a dent on the background of misery, but it is something—and in fact everything for the parents of that child. And it is infinitely better than increasing the misery. And soon small numbers add up. When I became involved in global health in the 1960s, more than 3 million children died each year because of the measles virus. Three million couples were added to the millions of others with an empty place at the table. Eventually, that number declined to 2 million, then 1 million, and now it is below 150,000. Still far too many but evidence of improvement.

Years ago, a tobacco executive from Rothmans in the United Kingdom was answering a question about how he could live with the idea of promoting smoking in Bangladesh. His response was that people didn't live long enough in Bangladesh to experience the adverse effects of tobacco, and, in addition, it was one of the few joys they could experience. The answer was appalling not only for its callousness but also for its ignorance.

People often look at life expectancy for a nation as the normal experience for everyone. They assume that if life expectancy in Ancient Greece was 35, for example, that that means 35 was old age in Greece. The truth is that any culture with high infant-mortality rates, in which 150 of every 1,000 babies born will die by their first birthday, will have a low life expectancy on average. But if a person makes it to reproductive age in that culture, he or she has a fair chance of living into their fifties or sixties. Many of the great historical figures in Greece lived into their seventies and beyond. Isocrates, for example, a great teacher of rhetoric, who stressed the ability to use language to address practical problems (and may be the father of liberal arts education), lived to age 99.

Therefore, a person in Bangladesh who lives long enough to take up smoking has that life shortened by tobacco. No matter how miserable life might be, it could only be made worse by a terrible final illness and by losing a spouse or a parent, as well as a means of support, earlier than necessary. Our job is to avoid premature mortality and unnecessary suffering.

So the perspective at the CDC was often one of minuscule efforts to bring some hope to miserable conditions. And somehow that situation bred humor. Perhaps in small ways, we were trying to bring light onto the very dark canvas we worked with. George Bernard Shaw was right when he said, "Life does not cease to be funny when people die, any more than it ceases to be serious when people laugh." It is the enjoyment of life that becomes our argument that life is worth all the trouble required. It gives a reason both to enjoy and to use our gifts for the improvement of other lives, so they may also enjoy it.

The CDC had plenty of humor. In staff meetings and in daily interactions, laughter was frequent. Dave Sencer was so competitive that any practical joke played on him required a response on his part. The first time he left me in charge of the CDC for a day when he was in Washington, DC, I left him a memo outlining some outlandish decisions supposedly made in his absence. One was a copy of a memo, with his signature, ostensibly sent to all CDC employees, outlawing the wearing of pantsuits at work. This was in the early days of this fashion statement, when women everywhere were enthusiastically embracing this custom. Sencer said nothing on his return, but the next day I had a call from his office asking if I could come down to discuss a problem.

As I entered his office, flashbulbs temporarily blinded me. When my sight returned, I saw that his entire office was filled with women in pantsuits.

I left for a backpacking trip with my family on the Pacific Crest Trail just before the Legionnaires' outbreak in Philadelphia. Because I had pulled a practical joke on Dave before leaving, my sons, knowing his usual way of reacting, were concerned that he would do something to us while camping. They wondered, around a campfire at night, if he would appear in a bear suit. On our descent from the mountains, we checked into a motel, and three of us went to a grocery store to buy food. On entering the store, totally unaware of the Legionnaires' outbreak unfolding in Philadelphia, the first thing we heard was the radio on the store speakers and Dave Sencer's voice, discussing the outbreak. But even before we knew the content of his discussion, one of my sons, recognizing his voice, said, "He found you, Dad."

The memorial service for Dave Sencer was held at the Emory School of Public Health. I shared a story that captured his wide knowledge, his quick response, and his wit:

I no longer remember the reason for the banquet. But I will never forget how Dave's humor caught me by surprise. For some reason the master of ceremonies began talking about Judges, chapter 15, verse 15. It is the story of Samson taking on the Philistines, picking up a jawbone and killing a thousand of them. It is not a story you casually insert into an introduction . . . unless, of course, you are introducing Samson . . . so there must have been a reason, but it is now lost to history. Dave got up, said thanks for the introduction and then, after recounting the passage as it is actually written, he added, "It is the first time that I have followed the jawbone of an ass." Try thinking of that without smiling.

Mohan Singh and the Making of Myth

The legend is that Hod Ogden, head of the CDC's health education programs, had just finished lunch in a place he would later describe as upscale (but that others in his group would describe as having woodchips and sawdust on the floor to absorb spilled drinks), when he picked a card out of the sawdust and read the name "Mohan Singh" on it. Hod said, "This is an interesting name, and he deserves to be known as a health educator." Mohan Singh is actually a common name, and famous people with that name have been scientists, poets, writers, and businessmen. For example, a Mohan Singh started the Oberoi Hotel chain.

But with Hod Ogden, the name became known in health education circles as a pundit. Eventually, two small books were published on the maxims of Mohan Singh, all originating in the mind of Hod Ogden (1,2). Hod had the temerity to actually quote Mohan Singh in some of his scientific publications, and it gradually became a game that he passed on to others. The quotes became famous in health education circles and continued to be found in health education books published in recent years. Evelyne de Leeuw

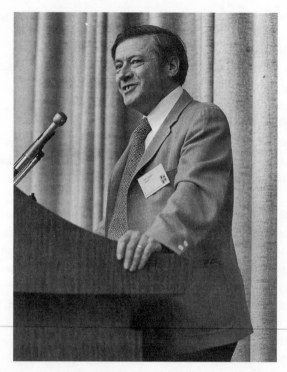

CDC health educator Hod Ogden, aka Mohan Singh, ca. 1973. Photo courtesy of David J. Sencer CDC Museum

has written about the impact felt in the early 1980s when she finally met the author of the maxims (3):

> During my university days I had studied, with great reverence, the proverbs of one Mohan Singh. To us, the sage Singh was the health education equivalent of the Dalai Lama. What transcendent wisdom, what lucid perspicacity, what cogent astuteness spoke from these pearls of profundity! And indeed, that evening in the Canadian capital, I was in the presence of Great Wisdom discovering that cutting-edge thought had nothing to do with physical age, and that Mohan Singh was Hod Ogden.

She went on to list some of her favorite Singh quotes:

He who lives by bread alone needs sex education.

Beware, lest the fragile lotus of health education be trampled by the elephants of reality.

Neither contemplation of the navel nor the writing of pamphlets can be shown to be cost-effective.

I would add:

Remember always to be grateful for the millions of people everywhere whose despicable habits make health education necessary.

The lotus, like health education, floats upon still waters; alas, while many admire their perfection, neither has visible means of support.

Consider the wombat . . . and be grateful.

The joy of wild rice is in the reaping: of wild oats, in the sowing.

As others picked up the idea from Ogden and used Mohan Singh quotes in their own scientific articles, the question became, "Could Singh," by now a mythical health educator,* "be quoted in all of the major medical journals?" The answer was yes. Never was he used to convey scientific information; always it was as philosopher, pundit, or health educator. A high point was reached when he was quoted in an editorial in the *New England Journal of Medicine* (4). This inspired Dave Sencer, on a trip to India, to send a letter to the editor, which he signed as Mohan Singh. His letter read, in part:

An American colleague has called my attention to the editorial article . . . Imagine my pride and wonderment in finding my humble words quoted so eloquently.

Unfortunately, however, in translating from the Telegu, there was a minor error, which I trust will not change the essence of the article. The quotation:

Seeing is not believing
Believing is not knowing
Knowing is not understanding
Understanding is not doing.

Should conclude:

Yet understanding can lead to doing . . .

M. Singh, M.B.B.S., B.S.Sc. (5)

---

*Each year, the American Public Health Association selects a member to receive the Mohan Singh Award for Humor, and a website of Mohan's sayings is maintained (http://ldb.org /mohan/maxim12.htm) in honor of Hod.

Fund-Raising Target

One year, as part of fund-raising for United Way, the CDC had a carnival in the parking lot with various attractions. I agreed to sit on a bench over a large tub of water while people threw a ball at a bull's-eye. If they hit it, I would be plunged into the water. I actually wasn't worried. After all, these were not professional pitchers, the target was relatively small, and the distance adequate for protection. However, I was amazed to see the long line of people this attraction drew. Many people who had never previously demonstrated their charitable instincts paid money to get baseballs to try their luck. I soon learned that falling in not only immersed me but also injured me each time I fell because the equipment was defective. The ball-throwing became frenzied. Although the target was small, apparently some had practiced for this opportunity to show their feelings. I fell no less than 100 times in three hours.

Another day, a group came requesting that I allow them to organize a roast of me. My first reaction was that it was not a good idea. However, when they indicated that they would charge admission and that the money would go for charity, I relented.

With little to work with, the staff exaggerated to make it truly a funny occasion. I was greatly concerned that night to see my current supervisors from Washington, DC, past supervisors, and dozens more lining up to show their considerable talent, heretofore hidden, in the art of ridicule. (Particularly memorable was Jim Curran's impersonation of me, carried off by wearing stilts.) In the end, all I could say was that I had agreed to this because of my interest in charity. If they didn't believe I had a strong commitment to charity, all they had to do was look at my immediate staff.

Retirement parties often involved a slapstick group called the "Hod Og players," named for Hod Ogden. The group would sing songs written about the retiree. The fear of such a sendoff had a very positive effect on the CDC roster. Many delayed their retirement dates, unwilling to endure the retirement party.

In meeting with people who worked at the CDC around 1980, the first reaction is always how much fun it was to be part of that organization. What a great legacy, to do important work and to have fun while doing it.

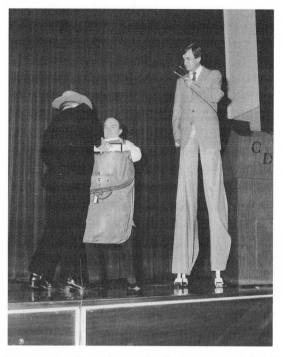

Dr. Jim Curran impersonating the author at a fund-raising roast, during his directorship of the CDC. Photo from Jim Curran.

Humor in a Tense International Meeting

Humor is often the social lubricant for meetings that are tedious, tiring or even tense. In 1967, while working in Eastern Nigeria, we were called to the then capital of Nigeria, Lagos, for a meeting to coordinate health educa-tion approaches. What should have been a routine meeting became tense for political reasons. The Eastern Region of Nigeria, with primarily Ibo workers, had jumped ahead in its smallpox eradication activities. This was annoying to members of other regions, including Yoruba tribe members from the Western Region. In addition, the political hostilities between the tribes were reaching a breaking point. The hostility was now being aimed at the health education materials presented by team members from the Eastern Region. The posters, pamphlets, and other materials were being ridiculed to the point that I was concerned the delegation from the Eastern Region might walk out.

But then Dr. Adetokunbo Lucas, a Yoruba and an esteemed professor from the University of Ibadan with a legendary sense of humor, said, "If we all agree that the first task of health education materials is to capture attention, it appears that the materials from the Eastern Region passed that test." No one else could have said that to make it humorous. But suddenly people were laughing at the obvious truth of the statement and the meeting settled into a productive discussion.

Global public health work can be difficult, frustrating, and intense. But it also rewarding and exhilarating. When levity is woven into our daily lives it improves *our* quality of life.

chapter 22

REDUCING THE TOLL OF INJURIES

During my years at the CDC, few public health areas were more frustrating than violence. The area is often divided into intentional and unintentional violence, although both facets have many common factors. Intentional violence is often seen as homicide, suicide, war, domestic abuse, and bullying. Unintentional violence is often considered as highway injuries, drowning, natural disasters, and occupational injuries. Both share certain risk factors, such as alcohol consumption or aggressive tendencies, and both can be reduced by changing the physical or psychological environment.

During my years as head of the CDC, we would annually include injury control in our budget requests, only to have the proposal rejected, accompanied by explanations that this topic involved highway safety, law enforcement, or some other area, but it was not a public health concern. Part of the problem may have been that the Public Health Service had a Division of Accident Prevention in the 1960s, which had moved to the National Highway Traffic Safety Administration. So there was little enthusiasm for trying to resurrect injury control at the CDC.

Highway safety experts had indeed shown the potential for prevention. Injuries and deaths per million miles driven had steadily declined in this country. Part of the reason was a change in the environment, including limited-access highways, banking of curves, relocating tail lights, seat belt use, airbags, and better headlights. Other reasons were driver education, campaigns against drinking and driving, campaigns to encourage and finally mandate seat belt use, and child restraints. Sometimes these changes were federal requirements, based on experience; at other times, they were the result of grassroots efforts. Today, child restraints are used for 99 percent of infants, and parents don't even question the requirement.

In the early 1970s, car injuries were the leading cause of death for young children in Tennessee when pediatrician Dr. Robert Sanders became chair of the state's chapter of the Accident Prevention Committee of the American Academy of Pediatrics. In 1976, Sanders proposed a state mandatory child-restraint law, which was defeated in committee. It is hard in retrospect to understand these political representatives, but they felt government should not interfere with parenting and even accused Sanders of having a financial interest in safety-seat manufacturing. He was persistent, however, and in 1978 the Tennessee Child Passenger Safety Law passed by two votes. Seven years later, all fifty states had passed similar laws without the matter ever going through Congress or the federal government. (Actually, almost all public health advances, whether coming from the states, as with child restraints, or coming from the federal government, as in many of the childhood vaccine initiatives, are based on demonstrations at local levels that an approach is feasible.)

Despite the lack of appropriations for an injury-control program, the CDC established the Violence Epidemiology Branch in 1983. This small group of two physicians, a sociologist, an anthropologist, and a statistician was asked to look at violence as a public health issue and to determine what could be done to save lives and preserve health.

The director for the program was an inspired choice. Mark Rosenberg, a former EIS officer, was well versed in epidemiology. He had returned to Boston from the CDC in Atlanta for a residency in psychiatry. He quickly brought the two disciplines of psychiatry and public health to a fruitful coalition bearing on injury as a public health problem.

Rosenberg was familiar with controversy. In 1975, while investigating a polluted water supply at Crater Lake in Oregon, he and other CDC investigators came under attack as "out-of-state bureaucrats who did not vote for Senator Hatfield." The investigators did not evoke a lot of sympathy from the folks in Oregon. He was to receive more such abuse in his new position.

It was not until after leaving the directorship of the CDC that I had an opportunity to be involved in a different approach to injury control. I was asked to chair an Institute of Medicine committee on the subject. Our goal was to make suggestions to improve the federal government's response to injury control.

It was a wonderful committee of people from the federal government, state and local governments, NGOs, and academia. After documenting the extent of the problem of injuries and death from violence, the committee sought a way to channel the federal interest. The committee sent a questionnaire to federal agencies that asked how much money they spent on injury control or injury research; it revealed sizable expenditures, often because research funding was included that was actually quite generic and tangential to the injury problem. This is the expected and often observed reaction as agencies position themselves in the hope that they will acquire resources if a new program is instituted.

A second questionnaire was sent to agencies that had reported significant involvement in injury control, asking them a similar question, but in a different way. If the federal government consolidated injury-control efforts, what would be their contribution to the consolidated program? Now, apparently worried that they might be asked to give up resources, these same agencies indicated that they were doing very little in injury control. As the committee reviewed possible places to focus the government's efforts, they reached the conclusion, after eliminating one place after another, to select the CDC—despite multiple arguments against that conclusion by myself and others. I was concerned that it would appear that I had engineered such a conclusion and, for that reason, argued against it, but the committee insisted on that result.

The IOM recommendation did not lead directly to a CDC program. HHS was still reluctant to make injury control or violence reduction a public health priority or responsibility. However, the committee was clear in its intent, choosing to title its report *Injury in America: A Continuing Public Health Problem* (1).

A declaration was not the same as funding, however. And, then, as happened so often during my time in public health, the unexpected happened. Congressman Bill Lehman from Florida had a deep interest in injury control and had come to know Mark Rosenberg. Lehman chaired the subcommittee that decided on appropriations for the Department of Transportation so he knew the impact of deliberate action on highway injuries and deaths. He included an item for $10 million in the budget of the Department of Transportation, *on the condition* that it would go to the CDC to establish a program on injury control. This is the kind of innovative government action that is so important and so rare. Many said they could not remember a similar maneuver. The money did go to the CDC to enhance the small injury research and control effort and brought renewed enthusiasm for a public health approach to injury control.

The year after receiving the $10 million from the Department of Transportation, there were high hopes that HHS would include injury in the CDC budget, but it did not. Congressman Lehman again placed it in the Department of Transportation budget. For three years, he had to take this approach until HHS conceded that this was a public health problem and should be funded by the Public Health Service. Bill Lehman should be added to the list of political heroes who changed the future of the health of the public.

The CDC set to work to carry out the objectives outlined by the Institute of Medicine of the National Academy of Sciences: to provide a scientific understanding of the causes of injuries and how they occur, to apply the findings from scientific studies to create programs to prevent injury, and to work in partnership with various groups dedicated to solving the injury problem in America. The program grew and provided better statistics, better analysis, and commonsense prevention ideas. As the program became stronger and covered larger areas of the injury landscape, the benefits became obvious. Thus, in 1992, it was officially made the Center for Injury Control.

Injury-control public health flourished. Academic centers worked on injury control, and research money became available. State health departments felt encouraged to support injury control. It was an optimistic time as the field became part of the great application of science to the improvement of human well-being.

The injury conversations led quite naturally to all areas of violence, which led to the question of what the possible role of a politically unbiased approach to gun safety could be. What if shooting incidents could be followed as one follows infectious diseases? Could a program collect and analyze the results as one would analyze a polio outbreak and discover ways of improving gun safety?

But it was too good to last. Public health absolutely needs the support of politicians. But it can also be totally undermined by the efforts of politicians and by forces more interested in turf or profit than health. Research on gun safety became a major political obsession.

After the 1994 election, there were many National Rifle Association-sponsored Internet postings, including one by a physician who wrote, "Goodbye CDC." It stated that a favorable makeup of Congress made it possible to stop the CDC gun research. The physician urged readers to contact their congressional representatives and even suggested that Dr. Rosenberg be investigated for possible illegal political lobbying.

Meanwhile, the NRA was pushing the same anti-CDC message through its powerful friends on Capitol Hill. On October 19, 1995, ten US senators, including majority whip Trent Lott and presidential candidate Bob Dole, wrote a "Dear Arlen" letter to Senator Arlen Specter, chairman of the Appropriations Subcommittee that oversaw HHS. It urged the elimination of the CDC's National Center for Injury Prevention and Control on the grounds that its work was wastefully "duplicative" and driven by "preordained political goals."

On May 1, 1996, Rep. Jay Dickey (R-Arkansas) grilled Mark Rosenberg at an appropriations hearing.

"Dr. Rosenberg," Dickey asked, "did you make the statement that you 'envision a long-term campaign similar to tobacco use and auto safety to convince Americans that guns are first and foremost a public health menace'"?

Actually, he did not, Rosenberg explained. The words were those of a journalist writing about public health research into gun violence. They did not even make logical sense, Rosenberg said. Obviously, he said, cars are not "first and foremost" a health menace. What he had said, "was that we don't even use the word 'gun control' and we don't think that you have to ban guns to prevent these injuries, the same way that we never had to ban cars but we saved hundreds of thousands of lives on the highway."

Rosenberg's explanations were not enough. In June, the House Appropriations Committee approved a Dickey amendment cutting $2.6 million out of the National Center for Injury Prevention and Control budget—the precise amount it was spending on firearms research of all kinds. The Senate eventually restored the money but earmarked it for traumatic brain injury surveillance.

This was not only a setback for the work at the CDC but also for states attempting to reduce firearm injuries and for ten research centers in academic institutions. The public health emphasis on sophisticated data collection "has been a major contribution [to public health]," said Philip Cook, a Duke economist who had been working on gun violence for a quarter of a century. "That was a great casualty of this cutback."

In 2013, Vice President Joe Biden headed an effort to find ways to improve gun safety after the horrendous tragedy of December 14, 2012, when twenty children and six adults were shot at the Sandy Hook Elementary School in Newtown, Connecticut. Some were outraged to find that the CDC had been prohibited from doing research on gun violence and wanted to know who was behind that action. It turned out to be Congress that was behind that action.

We are surrounded by enemies. Some are so small that they require microscopes to be seen. And some are in suits, occupying congressional offices or lobbying organizations, representing specific and special interests, rather than the interests of the public.

chapter 23

UNCOMMON PEOPLE

Science is the bedrock of public health, but people discover the truths of science and implement the knowledge to improve health. In the best of worlds, science would have the greatest role, and yet "tradition is the DNA of our beliefs," and, at times, our beliefs run roughshod over scientific fact. Our painfully slow response to global warming serves as an example. When we do get it right, it is usually a team effort. However, certain people stand out as characters, leaders, mentors, and problem solvers. Or, as problems. (Fortunately, space and good taste restrict the numbers that I will mention in that last category.)

C. Everett Koop could play all of those positive roles. When he was first nominated as surgeon general, there was quite an outcry from the public health community because he was a surgeon (which to me seemed quite appropriate for the title of surgeon general) and not a public health professional. I have never sympathized with that view because I believe public health is more philosophy and common sense than a specialty. Through the years, I have seen contributions made by people like Jim Grant, a lawyer by background and director of UNICEF in the 1980s or, more recently, Mary Selecky, a historian and Washington State health officer. So I approached Dr. Koop without prejudice.

Dr. Koop told me some years after his appointment that he dreaded his first visit to the CDC. The pro-life community regarded him as a hero, and they regarded the CDC as pariahs because we did abortion surveillance. That community never understood the difference between doing abortions and doing surveillance on the morbidity and mortality resulting from legal and illegal abortions. We were simply trying to document the complications and deaths from the practice. Dr. Koop was under pressure from his backers to close down our abortion surveillance program. He arrived at my office, and without others involved, we closed the door and sat at the conference table.

After the formalities, I said, "Dr. Koop, no matter what we talk about today we are both going to wonder when we will get to abortion. Why don't we start with that and get it out of the way?" When I finished my discussion of the topic, he was clearly overwhelmed by the logic of what we were doing, and he said, "If you weren't doing this I would have to start it. We simply have to know about the health impact of both legal and illegal abortions. How can I help?"

I told him I received hate messages each time we published the surveillance report. I asked if I could send him our abortion reports in draft so he could search for factual or scientific errors and find words or phrases that were red flags to be avoided. He agreed and followed through. We continued our important work, and the hate mail from the pro-life community stopped.

Our ability, with different backgrounds, to come together on the science, blossomed into a friendship of easy conversation and discussions beyond public health. Dr. Koop had a white beard and was often depicted by the press as looking like Abraham. He once told me of a significant donor to the Republican Party, who had decided that he actually *was* Abraham, she was Sarah, and they were destined to be together. She had now said she would have a press conference to announce that fact. Dr. Koop's question was whether I had any suggestions. I said perhaps, but first I must ask a delicate question. He asked, "What is that?" My reply, "Are you Abraham?"

Koop also taught me about delegating into the future. He called me one day when he was in his nineties and described a project that he could no longer attend to because of his age. He asked me whether I would carry it on for him, and I agreed. Koop taught me that careful delegation is a way to remain *scientifically active* after death.

Secretaries of HHS

In addition to Dr. Koop, I was fortunate in the people to whom I answered in the Public Health Service and the Department of Health and

Human Services (HHS). I worked directly for four different secretaries. The secretary of HHS provides the ultimate political support for CDC programs. The assistant secretary for health and the surgeon general provide scientific support, but without the support of the HHS secretary, important access to both Congress and the White House can be blocked.

Secretary Joseph Califano, the first of these, was extremely interested in health issues. Because he was so intent on changing the image of swine flu, I received his extra scrutiny. He actually sponsored the first influenza meeting in the new administration, a prerogative of the CDC in the past, and held the meeting in the Humphrey Building in Washington, DC, rather than at the CDC. He was so concerned about that first meeting that he sent a senior assistant to Atlanta to help me write my speech. The assistant did prepare a text, but I felt it was not usable and prepared my own speech. The meeting went well, and Califano loosened the reins.

Secretary Califano was absolutely superb in supporting programs. He decided we would greatly increase our immunization efforts, and he personally sought funds for this program. Once again his approach was to be involved directly, in this case by establishing an immunization office in Washington, DC, but he relaxed his control when he gained confidence in the CDC.

Califano could be demanding of subordinates, but they accepted this because of the support he provided. He would at times call me in the morning and ask me to be in Washington, DC, in the afternoon. On one occasion, I had just returned from Washington to the Atlanta airport when he paged me and asked me to take the next flight back to Washington.

I appreciated his ability to listen, see through issues, and then make a decision. On one occasion, deaths were reported in a small number of young children shortly after they received the diphtheria-tetanus-pertussis (DTP) vaccine. A limited number of vaccine lots were involved. Deaths in small healthy children are wrenching experiences. On initial investigation, the vaccines had no defects or unusual events in manufacturing, so the statisticians concluded that this was a random cluster occurrence with no vaccine implications. The immunization experts were concerned that any action to withdraw DTP vaccine might have the undesired effect of scaring people away from getting vaccinations.

Califano assembled the heads of all Public Health Service agencies as well as others in his office and had each person give his or her appraisal of the situation and recommendation. Every person said that Califano should explain to the public that this was a random grouping of sudden infant deaths, unrelated to vaccines. I was the second to the last person to speak and the first to give a contrary opinion. I worried that calling a cluster of deaths a statistical occurrence would not be understood and could even appear to be callous. I said that the conclusions were correct, as far as we could tell at the CDC, but that I would take a different approach. I suggested that he make the announcement as recommended but add that because of an abundance of caution an additional step would be taken. All lots of DTP vaccine that had been given to any infant who had suddenly died would be replaced with other vaccine lots; moreover, the Public Health Service would thoroughly review the records to make sure there had not been a manufacturing error overlooked in the initial investigation. My argument was that it gives the public more confidence to go overboard with caution than to appear cavalier. The last person to speak was Surgeon General Richmond, and the only thing he said was that he totally supported the last statement. Califano said he would consider all of our recommendations and ended the meeting. The next day he announced the department's approach—the recommendation that Richmond and I had made. That he would do this when only two people in the entire room supported it was gratifying. No vaccine problems were discovered even after an in-depth investigation.

Califano's support of the Public Health Service's antismoking activism was a decisive move that has resulted in major reductions in the shameful toll of death and disease due to tobacco.

Califano had asked me about my views regarding the role of the assistant secretary of health versus the surgeon general. I saw the assistant secretary of health as the line officer in charge of making policy and supervising the agencies. The surgeon general, on the other hand, was the senior officer of the Commissioned Corps—although not all public health service workers are in the corps. Indeed, the majority are civil servants. The surgeon general has a great bully pulpit but lacks the authority to direct or change programs. My suggestion was to have Richmond occupy both positions. It was a great solution and simplified life for many. But for obscure reasons, the practice was not followed in the future.

Richmond was a wonderful supervisor. A pediatrician by training, he had been a flight officer during World War II. He was cofounder of Head Start and a champion of mental health issues. The country was fortunate to have had Califano and Richmond during those years.

Secretary Patricia Harris moved from the US Department for Housing and Urban Development (HUD) to succeed Califano and brought an inquisitive mind to every problem. On my first meeting with her, I was asked to give a review of the CDC's activities. Things were going fine until I mentioned the number of children with elevated lead levels and the implications for mental impairment. I mentioned that lead in gasoline and lead in paint, particularly in urban dwellings, were the two largest sources for children's elevated lead levels. She stopped me, and said that her advisors at HUD had assured her that lead paint was not a hazard in city buildings. She threw up her hands dramatically and asked, "Who am I to believe?" I told her it might not always be the case, but in this instance, if I were her, I would believe me. She was taken aback for only a few seconds and then said, "I will do that, and you will bring me the proof."

It was the way she continued to operate. Give her the proof, and she would defend us to the end. As proof is the cornerstone of public health, this was a fantastic arrangement.

When President Reagan came to office, agency heads in the Public Health Service were fired. I received calls from other heads saying that they had received notice to be out of their offices by that afternoon. I began packing my office for the call that never came. Why wasn't I fired, too? Once again, I learned that we simply cannot see the future.

The reason I was spared actually went back to my first weeks as director of the CDC. At that time, I was told I had to meet with the senator from Pennsylvania, Richard Schweiker, to explain why his state had not been selected for a diabetes demonstration project. Senator Schweiker had engineered an appropriation for ten state demonstration programs to see what could be done to improve diabetes control. Now I had to explain why his state would not be in that number.

There are many gut-wrenching moments in public service. This was one of them. I made the appointment and told him the results. He asked how the selection had been made, and I walked him through the steps, including the use of outside reviewers, who had made the recommendations on which states should receive the money. He was unbelievably kind, and said he could find no fault with our approach, but he was sure that this would not happen to Pennsylvania again because he would personally be after them to provide a credible plan.

Periodically, after that meeting, I went to his office to brief him on the latest diabetes activities. On one occasion, he called to ask whether I could take his place in speaking to a diabetes dinner group as he had been asked to go to the White House that night. I now realized he trusted me, and trust is the glue for partnerships and coalitions. I did give the talk for him, but it is not pleasant to be the substitute speaker when people are expecting a senator. In later years, I would experience the same disappointment when I would substitute for President Carter. I would tell the audience that it is like being the brother of Jesus with people saying to me, "Why can't you be more like your brother?"

The next day, I heard that President Reagan had asked Senator Schweiker to be the new secretary of HHS, and the call to step down as the CDC director did not come.

The final secretary during my time was Secretary Margaret Heckler. I had less contact with her than with my other supervisors. She did not seem deeply interested in the CDC or in health.

Ed Brandt

During the Reagan years, the assistant secretary for health (my immediate boss) was Dr. Ed Brandt. In the mold of Richmond, it would be hard to imagine a better informed and involved supervisor. He had a medical degree and a PhD in biostatistics. He also had a theology degree and straddled the worlds of science and ethics with comfort.

It would have been a mistake to try and fool Brandt with probabilities or standard deviations. On one occasion, he interrupted a talk I was giving to protest a statement that I had just made, the first time I had ever cited that particular fact. I had said that the life expectancy of the average American had increased by seven hours a day since January 1, 1900. He said that could not possibly be true. At the end of my presentation, he apologized to the audience for interrupting but said that the figure had stunned him and while I was speaking he had done his own calculations. His conclusion was that I was in fact wrong. It was not an increase of seven hours a day but an increase of seven hours and six minutes a day!

Art Buchwald

He wasn't a politician or a public servant, but this famous American humorist was a stinging political satirist in his syndicated column for the *Washington Post*. I met Buchwald by chance alone. One day, I boarded the plane for the return trip from Washington, DC, to Atlanta and recognized Buchwald, already seated. His newspaper columns were always entertaining in a Mark Twain sort of way. I recall a column in which he was making fun of the executive branch. The next day, he had an irate call from the State Department complaining that the Soviets had found it so amusing that

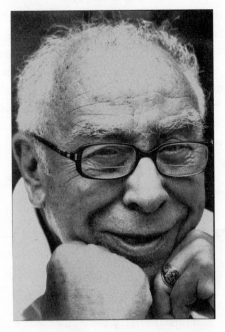

Art Buchwald. Photo by Mark Lovewell, courtesy of the *Vineyard Gazette*

they had reprinted it in *Pravda*. The State Department said they did not want that sort of publicity. Buchwald's response was, "Stop them."

I ignore celebrities so as not to invade their privacy but was surprised when Buchwald moved to an empty seat next to me after the plane door closed. He was sociable and wanted to talk. He asked about my family and related funny stories to tie into each piece of information. He was going on to Texas but got off in Atlanta, simply to keep talking until his plane was ready to depart.

I asked him whether he ever gave pro bono speeches, and soon he agreed to come to the CDC and entertain us free of charge. On the day selected, he had a family medical problem to deal with but still arrived, as he said he would, and provided an absolutely riveting and funny evening of entertainment.

A year later the *Journal of the American Medical Association* asked whether I could convince Buchwald to write an editorial on the role of humor in healing. I called his office, and his secretary said he was at the hospital with his wife, who was in serious condition. But his secretary relayed the request, and in the midst of his own grieving process he wrote the editorial.

The final story concerns an invitation we both had to be on a panel at the University of Minnesota. After I had agreed to go, President Carter asked me to go to Sudan, where we were seeking an extension of a peace interlude to do medical work. I told President Carter I would do that if he would explain to Art Buchwald why I couldn't join him for the dinner and panel. President Carter did that, and Art Buchwald said, "All things considered, I suppose I would prefer a call from a president to dinner with Bill Foege!" But then, to my complete surprise, he donated his $30,000 speaking fee for a scholarship in my name. It provides support of about $1,500 each year for a public health student, and I receive information on the recipient.

Other Gifted People

Now I recognize my inability to do justice to dozens, even hundreds, of gifted people who impressed me during the CDC years, and so I surrender in my hope of describing a few who inspired me.

Jim Grant, a lawyer, became an exceptional director of UNICEF and pulled people and resources into the attempt to make life better for children around the world.

Halfdan Mahler, a minister's son from Denmark, brought compassion and soaring rhetoric to the almost impossible job of coordinating a global approach to the improvement of health, with special attention to the poor.

Peter Bell, another lawyer, was passionate about improving the lives of the disenfranchised and left Califano's staff to work with NGOs and eventually became head of CARE.

Andrew Young, a minister, went from being the voice of reason who could bridge the racial divide during the civil rights revolution to becoming our UN ambassador. He could also be counted on to bridge nationalities, becoming the ambassador of the developing world to the United States.

Maynard Jackson, a lawyer and brother of a public health worker, became mayor of Atlanta and a constant supporter of the CDC.

John Lewis, the symbol of nonviolence in action during marches and riots in the South in the 1960s, would become involved in various civil rights efforts. President Carter named him as associate head of ACTION, a government program responsible for running the Vista program, the Retired Senior Volunteer Program, and the Foster Grandparent Program, before he was elected to Congress. He responded to every request for help in public health over decades.

And it was during the CDC years that I met President and Mrs. Carter. They are both persons of such quality and accomplishment that justice to their contributions is only possible in a future book.

This is an impoverished list, knowing as I do how many uncommon people have influenced my life. Please see the appendix for a fuller list.

chapter 24

AIDS

Overwhelming Public Health

It is a merciful God who doesn't allow us to see the future.
—Brendon Phibbs, World War II surgeon, *The Other Side of Time* (1987)

For decades, the public health community has faced previously unknown diseases—on average, a new one every year. Legionnaires' disease, Ebola virus, Lassa fever, green monkey disease, toxic shock—the list continues. The first cases of AIDS might have been simply one more addition to that list but for two things. First, it was not the discovery of an old, but previously unrecognized, disease. AIDS turned out to be a new human disease. Second, the outbreak was not limited or small. It became a pandemic that shook the foundations of public health, science, immunology, economics, development, and politics—indeed, all of society.

Many have told this story. This is not an attempt to document AIDS but rather to tell a few of the stories I observed personally.

The beginning was muted: an *MMWR* report on June 5, 1981, of five men who had been treated for *Pneumocystis carinii* pneumonia (1). All of these cases were laboratory confirmed, and two were fatal. This was an unusual diagnosis for young, healthy people. The only link seemed to be that they were gay.

Within days of the *MMWR* publication, reports came in from other hospitals of a similar disease. New York City and San Francisco were especially involved, and the spectrum became clearer. The patients were suffering from a variety of opportunistic infections as the result of a compromised immune system. This was a disease that was attacking the immune system, the traditional defense mechanism our bodies use to protect us from foreign organisms. In addition, some of the patients were suffering from Kaposi's sarcoma, a tumor known in Africa but relatively rare in this country.

The CDC response was unprecedented, and Paul Wiesner, director of the Sexually Transmitted Disease Program, was one of its heroes. He immediately assigned investigators to characterize and understand the new syndrome. The ensuing investigation quickly surpassed what the CDC had invested in the Legionnaires' disease investigation five years earlier. I mention this because later some accused the government of responding slowly because the patients were predominantly homosexuals. The erroneous conclusion that we had responded slowly was based on following budget figures without realizing that it takes some years for the authorization and appropriation of funds for new projects to become obvious in budget documents. What the CDC did is what it has always done with a newly recognized disease: use existing budget lines in the offices of epidemiology, venereal diseases, laboratory sciences, and the EIS.

As these CDC investigators became immersed in the outbreak, they had no idea of the magnitude of suffering and death about to be revealed. They had no idea it would take several years to release a definitive statement on prevention of this disease, that it would be shown to be a virus that infected with some efficiency, that it had a remarkably long incubation period, and that it would contaminate the blood supply of health facilities around the world. Nor could CDC investigators know then that it would take two decades to develop therapy and three decades to see the first cure. A third of a century later, there is still no vaccine. CDC AIDS investigators also could not know then that for some of them it would be the focus of their entire professional lives. No one would have imagined almost 600,000 Americans dying—and another 1.2 million infected—in the next thirty years from this disease.

A second hero, Dr. Jim Curran, was appointed as the head of a unit focusing exclusively on the new entity. He was blessed with a deputy, Dr. Harold Jaffe, who was unflappable in his pursuit of truth.

The opportunistic infections AIDS patients were exhibiting made sense if the patients had a compromised immune system. The occurrence of Kaposi's sarcoma was different. This is a tumor characterized by nodules, bumps, or raised portions that might be red, purple, brown, or black. They are found on the skin but spread to the mouth and gastrointestinal and respiratory tracts. They can be slow growing or explosive in growth. They cause physical and mental suffering and often progress to death.

Because Kaposi's sarcoma did not fit into the category of opportunistic infections and was thus puzzling, Curran organized a Kaposi's Sarcoma and Opportunistic Infections Task Force in 1981 to explore what was known about this condition. Clarity was not apparent for thirteen years, until 1994, when a viral cause was discovered for the condition. Only then could it be seen that it fit with other opportunistic conditions, made worse with a compromised immune system.

The Kaposi's task force involved the most prominent investigators of this rare condition from around the world. I had been taught in medical school to put the accent on the "o" in pronouncing Kaposi and so that is how I pronounced it when welcoming the group and thanking them for the service they were about to give. When I finished, one participant said we should start by getting the pronunciation correct. He said it was pronounced with the emphasis on the first syllable, the Kap. He went on to say that Dr. Kaposi actually pronounced it KA'-pa-she, but that it did not really matter since his name was actually Cohen. While some stories say he changed his name to hide his Jewish origins to gain admission to the University of Vienna, he told a different story. He said he changed his name to avoid confusion with five other Cohen faculty members. In any case, he first described the condition in 1872.

Curran and his team were overwhelmed. The numbers of AIDS cases continued to grow, and it became increasingly clear this was a fatal disease. It was a shock to face the fact that all patients might die once symptoms began. The team quickly developed case definitions and modified the definitions as more information became available. The CDC summarized the findings on an ongoing basis and predicted that the clinical cases identified were a small tip of a very large iceberg.

Within a year of the first report, the *MMWR* carried an article of a cluster of nineteen cases in Los Angeles (2). It became clearer that sexual transmission between gay men was a significant route of transmission of this agent. Although no agent had been identified, investigators were increasingly certain that they were dealing with a virus.

By August 1983, the task force was comfortable in publishing what they knew about risk factors. A case-control study of gay men with Kaposi's or *Pneumocystis* pneumonia, as compared to gay men without the disease, showed risk factors included a larger number of male sex partners (median of 61 per year versus 27 for controls), contact with feces during sex, and a higher incidence of syphilis and hepatitis. The findings were published in the *Annals of Internal Medicine* in August 1983 (3). A March 1984 diagram of

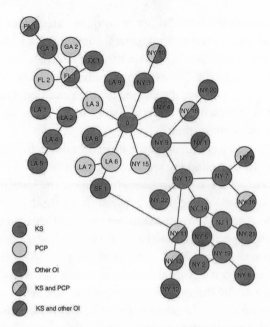

Sexual contacts among homosexual men with AIDS. *Circle*=AIDS patient. *Lines connecting circles*=sexual exposures. Indicated city or state is place of residence of a patient at the time of diagnosis (FL=Florida; GA=Georgia; LA=Los Angeles; NJ=New Jersey; NY=New York; PA=Pennsylvania; SF=San Francisco; TX=Texas). Abbreviations: 0=patient zero (described in text); KS=Kaposi's sarcoma; OI=opportunistic infection; PCP=*Pneumocystis* pneumonia. Redrawn from 1984 *American Journal of Medicine*

sexual contact between cases showed a remarkable amount of spread of this disease from a single index case (4).

While the investigators were increasingly convinced of a viral cause of the disease, some were concerned this might be a toxin, an environmental agent, or the result of drug use by patients. The above pictorial provided a strong case for an infectious agent that moved quickly between geographic locations.

Every day seemed to bring more sad news on numbers involved, potential dangers in transmission, and the frightening lethality of the disease. One of the hardest days was when it became clear that the agent was spreading to patients with hemophilia A. This group had a history of heartache best known because of European royalty afflicted with the condition. It is caused by an X-linked recessive gene that results in bleeding due to insufficient factor VIII production, usually in males. Factor VIII is an important ingredient in the clotting mechanism. In those with insufficient factor VIII, minor bumps and bruises may lead to serious problems, such as bleeding into joints. Internal bleeding was a frequent cause of death.

Until the twentieth century, little could be done for these patients. (The cause of the disease was thought to be fragile blood vessels, rather than a clotting defect.) In 1937, two doctors, Patek and Taylor, found that they could control the bleeding by giving a substance they isolated from the plasma of other people. In the 1950s, whole blood was often used. By the 1960s, however, Judith Pool had discovered a way to precipitate factor VIII from plasma. For the first time, large numbers of patients could be treated to prevent bleeding. Soon a freeze-dried product revolutionized treatment.

The problem was that the products were derived from pools of plasma collected from large numbers of donors. Anywhere from 1,000 to many thousands of donors contributed to each lot of factor VIII. It would not take much to contaminate the entire supply of factor VIII. Hemophiliacs would die without the administration of factor VIII, but now it was clear they could also die if they took factor VIII.

Until this time, arguments still raged on the cause of AIDS. With the diagnosis of AIDS in hemophiliacs, CDC investigators were convinced this was a virus.

The CDC summarized information on the first three hemophilia cases in the July 16, 1982, *MMWR* (5) a little over a year after the first AIDS article. At the beginning of that week, a conference sponsored by the Mt. Sinai School of Medicine was held in New York City. This was to be a chance for all the various theories on the origin of AIDS to be presented, although the main debate would be on whether it was a virus or a toxin. Jim Curran and I attended that meeting and presented the CDC findings on patients with hemophilia. Jim recalls that as a memorable point in the virus story because the other theories on the origin of the disease lost much of their credibility with that finding.

Scientists, of course, often have different perspectives. However, a system exists for following evidence, and soon most scientists reach agreement. But not all. Peter Duesberg, at the University of California, Berkeley, has consistently denied that HIV is the cause of AIDS. He sees HIV as a harmless virus and the real problem as long-term drug use and the use of antiretroviral drugs. Reviewers of his articles concluded he had a right to dissent but that he was selective in the use of literature and therefore his opinion was not credible.

Usually such dissent is valuable because it causes others to relook at their conclusions. Sometimes it can be deadly. When Duesberg served on an advisory panel to President Thabo Mbeki of South Africa, it resulted in a disaster in that country, as Mbeki failed to provide antiretroviral drugs and thousands of South Africans died of AIDS. It is a sobering reminder to all that there are consequences to misunderstanding and misjudging science. In clinical medicine, one way to redress errors is through malpractice procedures. Public health and political malpractice lack an effective corrective approach. The result is that blatant malpractice is excused as a difference of opinion.

As soon as the CDC had identified the risk to persons with hemophilia, we knew blood transfusions would pose a problem. It came to pass, but, as with factor VIII, we had no way to screen blood donors. Initial efforts at protecting the blood supply were aimed at discouraging donors in high-risk groups. Gay men were in that group, but a higher-than-expected incidence of AIDS had also been shown in people from Haiti. There was considerable pushback from the gay community and from Haitian political leaders to this recommendation. Even the blood banks were reluctant to implement such policies.

On March 4, 1983, before a virus had been isolated, a landmark article was published in the *MMWR*. It was entitled "Prevention of Acquired Immune Deficiency Syndrome (AIDS): Report of Interagency Recommendations" (6). What is remarkable is that without the isolation of a virus, the report showed the power of epidemiology. It provided information on the risk factors associated with sexual practices and the risk of contact with body fluids. Indeed, it contained sufficient information to actually stop the AIDS epidemic if it would be possible to alter human behavior. But that task proved too difficult.

Conclusions in the article (6):

1. Sexual contact should be avoided with persons known or suspected to have AIDS. Members of high-risk groups should be aware that multiple sexual partners increase the probability of developing AIDS.

2. As a temporary measure, members of groups at increased risk for AIDS should refrain from donating plasma and/or blood. This recommendation includes all individuals belonging to such groups, even though many individuals are at little risk of AIDS. Centers collecting plasma and/or blood should inform potential donors of this recommendation. The Food and Drug Administration (FDA) is preparing new recommendations for manufacturers of plasma derivatives and for establishments collecting plasma or blood. This is an interim measure to protect recipients of blood products and blood until specific laboratory tests are available.

3. Studies should be conducted to evaluate screening procedures for their effectiveness in identifying and excluding plasma and blood with a high probability of transmitting AIDS. These procedures should include specific laboratory tests as well as careful histories and physical examinations.

Two years after the first reports, thousands of cases of AIDS had been reported in the United States, and the best guesses were that this disease was caused by a virus spread through sexual activity, especially by gay men, and by exposure to body fluids, including blood products. It was to be a year before a virus was isolated and reported in the literature. Yet solid public health work had already identified the prevention procedures required.

The Pasteur Institute Discovers the AIDS Virus

Science was rapidly closing in on finding the virus involved. The Pasteur Institute in Paris underwent an expansion in 1972 to include a new unit for the study of viruses that cause cancer. Luc Montagnier became the director, and soon after the first reports, he found himself focused on finding the virus that caused AIDS. By the fall of 1982, some of the scientists working with the institute had become convinced that AIDS was caused by a virus of African origin that infected T-4 cells. On October 5, 1982, Jacques Leibowitch from Raymond Poincaré University Hospital gave a seminar on the "Retroviral Hypothesis in AIDS."

Meanwhile, at NIH in the United States, the lab of Robert Gallo had been working on a virus called human T-cell lymphotropic virus (HTLV), types I and II. These were known to cause cancers in humans, and there was speculation that they were also involved with AIDS.

It was clear there was a race between NIH and the Pasteur Institute regarding which one would be first to isolate a virus. On February 2, 1983, Montagnier had a letter hand-carried to Robert Gallo at NIH regarding his finding of a virus, which they later found to be different from the virus isolated by Gallo. Montagnier's group published their results on May 20, 1983, in *Science* (7). Great confusion persisted regarding Gallo's HTLV-I and II viruses and whether they were the same as the French virus. A September meeting at Cold Spring Harbor, New York, attempted to sort out the issue, but US researchers were scornful of the French results. The proceedings, published nine months later, described an HTLV-III virus that had not been mentioned at the meeting itself. After the fact, a new virus was being introduced from NIH. Could this be an independent isolation of an AIDS virus? Had the two labs finished the race in a dead heat with both having isolated the new virus?

In early 1984, a virologist shared with me his belief that the HTLV-III virus isolated by the Americans was actually Montagnier's virus. Having no way to confirm this myself, I took the information to my supervisor, Dr. Ed Brandt, assistant secretary of health in the Public Health Service. His response was that he would see what he could learn but not to worry. His comment was, "Science ultimately settles these issues."

On April 24, 1984, shortly after I left as director of the CDC, the secretary of Health and Human Services, Margaret Heckler, held a press conference with Ed Brandt, Robert Gallo, and others to announce that scientists at NIH had isolated the AIDS virus, the HTLV-III virus. She added that they would soon have a test for testing blood products and within two years federal laboratories would produce a vaccine. Gallo described his new virus in the May 4, 1984, issue of *Science* (8).

In December 1983, the Pasteur Institute applied for a US patent for a diagnostic kit based on the French virus. Five months later, NIH applied for a patent for Gallo's AIDS diagnostic kit. This NIH patent was issued a year later, while the Pasteur Institute was still waiting for its patent. NIH could now receive income from the use of its diagnostic kits.

The AIDS virus changes so quickly that significant variations are seen in the virus even as the virus spreads from one patient to the next. Yet later analysis found the NIH HTLV-III virus and the French virus to be essentially identical. My informant had been correct. The conclusion of many was that the NIH HTLV-III strain might have been accidentally grown from the French virus.

To fast-forward, in 2008, Luc Montagnier and Françoise Barré-Sinoussi were awarded the Nobel Prize in Physiology or Medicine for discovery of the AIDS virus. Ed Brandt was correct that science will eventually sort out these difficulties.

Jim Curran turned out to be a master at dealing with various groups. He was comfortable working with basic scientists and quickly learned their vocabulary. He was comfortable with clinicians, having spent time as one. And he was comfortable with academics. But perhaps most important, he was comfortable with patients and the gay community. The latter was frustrated with the pace of the scientific response to AIDS, perhaps not realizing how different this organism was from any previously encountered and understandably suspicious of a government that had always made them feel second class. And they were watching their friends die. Many became bitter.

Some became militant and shrill in their demands. But somehow Jim Curran did not lose his way, and the gay community began to trust him.

AIDS in Africa: A "Radio Disease"

The next disconcerting development was the rapid spread of AIDS in Africa and other countries around the world. In Africa, the disease was spread through heterosexual contact in most cases, and it spread with awesome speed. As in the United States, a risk factor was an increased number of sexual partners. In Africa, success in most fields led to increased wealth and the means of paying for or attracting many sexual partners. Therefore, young successful men appeared to have higher rates of both partners and HIV than less affluent men. The professions were becoming decimated. It was difficult to produce teachers, medical personnel, church workers, pilots, or others fast enough to refill the gaps left by those who were dying.

But the most crucial factor in Africa came down to the lack of power for women. A cursory look might give a different impression. The casual observer sees that women do the farmwork, gather wood for cooking, cook, work and trade in markets, and get children ready for school. Women appear to be the backbone of the society. But these tasks describe who does the work, not who has the power.

This lack of power extends to decisions on sex. Women often have no power in determining when they will have sex. They often have no power to insist on faithfulness, and they are often coerced into sex. Likewise, young women often need to trade sexual favors simply to get school fees. Prostitutes have difficulty insisting on the use of condoms, or they will not get a customer. Women's lack of power has fueled the AIDS epidemic in Africa.

African countries also found it difficult to admit the numbers of cases they were seeing lest it hurt tourism. The 1980s and 1990s were times of severe depression in African health. All of the gains in immunization and reductions in infant mortality and deaths from other diseases seemed to be mocked by the increased deaths and suffering from AIDS.

In 1987, Dr. Seth Berkley, supported by a Rockefeller Foundation grant, was working in Uganda on child health projects for the Task Force for Child Survival. He sent a letter saying that he had just completed an analysis of HIV rates in pregnant women in prenatal clinics in Uganda and was documenting an alarming increase. He asked if he could get permission to pursue this problem. The Task Force for Child Survival, which I now directed, urged him to do so.

A year later, in August 1988, President Carter was scheduled to visit Uganda. President Museveni, the head of state, asked for briefings from various people as part of his preparation for the meeting. Dr. Berkley briefed him on a variety of topics and, in the process, showed him the graph on the increase in HIV rates in pregnant women. The numbers seemed to be increasing almost by the month. President Museveni was shocked but said, "If I know this, everyone should know it." He proceeded to share the information and even had the graph published. This was the beginning of transparency in African countries, allowing them freedom to report the truth about AIDS.

India was not experiencing the same numbers of AIDS cases as Africa, at least if one could believe the reports. One day, Vulimiri Ramalingaswami, a friend for many years and one of the most revered scientists in India, sought my advice. He said he had been asked to suggest a response for India if it were to have a problem with AIDS. He asked for suggestions. I replied, as I had often in public health cases, that we should figure out first how to get to the truth. My suggestion was to test prostitutes on the New Delhi to Calcutta highway. He looked absolutely startled and asked me what I knew. I knew nothing, but said I would start with the places I expected the virus would first appear, and based on African experience, prostitutes and truck drivers were a potent opportunity for virus transmission. He then confided that the reason he was being asked for a plan was that a small sample of prostitutes on that very highway had already tested positive for AIDS.

In India, as in Africa, AIDS spread quickly from the population of sex workers, to truck drivers, to the wives of truck drivers, and then into the general population.

Dr. Seth Berkley later worked with AIDS for the Rockefeller Foundation. He and the foundation concluded that the ultimate answer to the problem would be a preventive vaccine. Although the difficulties were far greater than implied by Margaret Heckler's announcement that a vaccine would be developed in two years, the Rockefeller Foundation, with a grant of $10 million, started the International AIDS Vaccine Institute (IAVI). Dr. Berkley became the president. The Gates Foundation had great confidence in the Rockefeller Foundation and later pledged $100 million to IAVI. The institute organized incredible scientific efforts that helped elucidate how the virus operated and subdued the immune system response.

Some were concerned that the Gates grant would cause others to withhold vaccine development funds; the argument was that the Gates Foundation would now be the chief funder. But that is not the way people operate. An informant at NIH told me (although he said he would always deny the story if asked) that NIH scientists held a meeting after the Gates grant was announced. They concluded that they could not afford to have an outside funder solve the problem of an AIDS vaccine, and they asked what it would take to make sure NIH stayed in the lead for developing the vaccine. This led to a more robust program at NIH than would have developed in the absence of the Gates grant. Research is augmented by competition, and developments have been faster than if Rockefeller and Gates had not entered the field.

Upon leaving the CDC, I went to the Carter Center, where the Carters had embraced global health programs in immunization, mental health, Guinea worm eradication, trachoma, onchocerciasis (river blindness), and agriculture and its impact on nutrition, as well as their work in democracy and free elections. While there, the executive director of AID Atlanta, Sandy Thurman, and her coworker Nancy Paris, asked me whether I would become chair of the AID Atlanta board. This suddenly gave me experience with AIDS at the ground level. The courage of these young men who continued to work at improving social services and support activities for others as they faced their own death sentence was both inspiring and depressing.

A year after beginning the work with AID Atlanta, I found myself in an uncomfortable social situation with community leaders that included stories at the expense of the gay community. I felt compelled to share my experience and asked the group what it was that so scared the straight community? Furthermore, did anyone actually think being gay was a choice? Observing the prejudice expressed by society, why would people choose that position? My opinion was that people were gay because of genetics, and that attempts to live in opposition to one's genetics led to even more discomfort than if persons were open about their sexual preferences. It escaped my understanding how people could be so confident of their views that they would torment others.

At any rate, the experience of working with AIDS-infected persons was profound. Human nature is baffling, and how people under the same threat of the virus can fail to embrace one another is one of those mysteries. But the conflict between the gay community and the black community has continued to fester throughout the AIDS epidemic.

Good news and bad news continued to alternate. In 1987, the first drugs capable of inhibiting HIV appeared. The virus requires reverse transcriptase to replicate, and these new drugs inhibited this essential protein. The drugs did not cure the disease but made AIDS a truly chronic disease.

In a sense, AIDS already *was* a chronic disease. The immune system was almost, but not quite, capable of stopping the infection. This determined virus would produce billions of new viruses every day; the immune system would attack and disable almost that number every day. But the immune system was just shy of being a match for HIV. Over the days, weeks, and months, virus production would slowly exceed virus destruction. In a healthy person, it might take five years, ten years, or even fifteen years before the immune system had to acknowledge it simply could not keep up, and the virus would slowly take over the body. The reverse-transcriptase inhibitors made the contest more even, and the virus could not overwhelm the immune system. What had been a chronic disease over a decade might change into a chronic disease over many decades.

But resistance to the new drug was likely to develop. Fortunately, in 1995, protease inhibitors became available. These antiviral drugs also inhibited an essential protein. Combining the two inhibitors provided another boost to a patient's immune system. Two years later, a different type of reverse-transcriptase inhibitor became available. In 2003, a fourth new drug became available to inhibit entry of the virus into cells. And in 2007, integrase inhibitors provided an additional attack on virus multiplication.

Initially, it appeared that these medications were simply too expensive to be used in the developing world, but the George W. Bush administration made a commitment to provide funds to greatly increase treatment in poor countries. It has changed the course of history. An increasing percentage of AIDS patients around the world are being treated and that has reduced the amount of virus circulating in treated people. This decreases their ability to transmit the infection to others. Patients have returned to work, and family structures again have a chance to be repaired. This is a positive and long-lasting legacy of President George W. Bush.

The science will advance. Human foibles remain. Treatment is a stopgap measure. The real answer to AIDS is to stop transmission of the virus rather than to attack it patient by patient. Work on a vaccine must continue. Prevention must be enhanced. The treatment of AIDS patients would seem to be a wonderful place to start with massive education programs on how to avoid transmission; promoting condoms for every sexual encounter; delaying sexual activity; and positive incentives, such as educational opportunities for young people. Instead, in most countries, treatment has consumed public health people and resources, and the focus on prevention is lost.

A second foible has been the elevation of religious beliefs to thwart good science. The US PEPFAR (President's Emergency Plan for AIDS Relief) program emphasized abstinence and fidelity and discouraged condom use. No one can fault the first two, but human experience is that to discourage condoms is simply to wish that people were as good as you want them to be. Wishes do not protect the wives of men who have sex outside of marriage without using condoms. Hopes do not prevent a child from becoming an orphan because their father did not use a condom.

I went to hear the head of PEPFAR when he spoke in Seattle, Washington. I was impressed by his zeal, his grasp of managerial issues, and his desire to improve the world. But he was unyielding in his emphasis on fidelity, abstinence, and unavailability of condoms. I was surprised later to learn he was stepping down. Days later I learned that his name had been found on the D.C. Madam's list.

This was certainly a step back from the years of Dr. C. Everett Koop. He became surgeon general under President Reagan with great fanfare from the religious right because of his strong stand on abortion. But Dr. Koop became an enigma for the Republican Party because he listened to science. He became a supporter of the AIDS program when others in the administration wanted to punish the victims. He listened before making up his mind.

Two final stories. In January 2000, while new drugs were changing the outlook for AIDS in the United States, the future was bleak for Africa. I was now working with the Bill & Melinda Gates Foundation, and it hosted a meeting in Seattle in January 2000 to discuss AIDS with other foundations. The question was whether we collectively could see a way forward that warranted investments by these foundations.

Some background to the meeting is important. In 1987, Merck's chief executive officer, Dr. Roy Vagelos, had offered the drug Mectizan for the treatment of onchocerciasis. He had asked the Task Force for Child Survival to administer the program against river blindness, and it had been a great success. At the twenty-fifth anniversary celebration, in October 2012, the company reported that it had given 1 billion free treatments of Mectizan for the program in Africa and Central America.

A decade after the launch of that program, the successor to Vagelos, Ray Gilmartin, asked a small group to advise the company on AIDS. He said Merck was so pleased with the outcome of the Mectizan program that it now wanted to see how it could help with AIDS. The group advised Merck to avoid piecemeal approaches but rather to ask the question of how modern science could be applied under African conditions of high disease rates, malnutrition, urban crowding, and poverty to solve AIDS problems. In late 1999, the group was called back to see the results. Guy Macdonald of Merck had developed a comprehensive plan that was exciting. I asked him to present his plan to the Seattle AIDS meeting, and he agreed.

The day before the meeting was to start, the group planning the meeting learned that I had invited Dr. Macdonald to present, and they absolutely refused to allow it on the basis that a for-profit company would have commercial interests and would likely have little to offer. Knowing Macdonald was already on a plane, I pressed the case, arguing that it could not possibly hurt us to hear the perspective of a corporation that had examined closely what could be done. After hours of debate, the group capitulated as a favor to me. The next day Guy Macdonald made a stunning presentation. It made them bolder in developing possible approaches.

At the end of the second day, the group had decided on six ideas to pursue that provided some possibilities for "light at the end of the long, dark AIDS tunnel" in developing countries. Each foundation agreed to pursue what it could, and I was asked to present the six ideas to Bill Gates for possible support from his foundation.

The meeting with Bill Gates did not start well. He first wanted to discuss a grant proposal that had been sent to him that seemed to encapsulate every problem that he wanted to avoid in the future. He told us that he was not interested in proposals that involved bottomless pits, especially when it would be hard to measure progress. He did not want to obligate the foundation to do things that should be done by government and other groups. He was reluctant to invest in projects that, once started, would require continuing support, perhaps for a long time.

As he continued to enumerate the things he did not want to see, it struck me that all of them were part of the six proposals I wanted to discuss. In addition, the AIDS arena would be a new area for the Gates Foundation, with many implications.

But my lack of flexibility destined me to describe the meeting on AIDS with the six specific proposals that had resulted. I had gone through the first five proposals when he suddenly stopped me to ask how much money we were proposing. I told him that our first estimate was $50 million a year for ten years. His immediate response was, "It will take a lot more than that!" With that, I was emboldened to go to idea number six, which had to do with AIDS orphans in Africa. If anything was a bottomless pit with implications for future funding, this was it. His response was, "You can't worry about AIDS in Africa without worrying about the orphans." He told us to proceed with all six ideas. This eventually led to the recruitment of Merck in a collaborative program in Botswana, the recruitment of Helene Gayle from the CDC, microbicide efforts, the Hope for African Children Initiative (HACI), and other AIDS projects.

On the way back to our foundation offices, I asked Bill Gates Sr.—Bill's father, a lawyer, and the first president of the Gates Foundation—to help me understand what the two of us had just witnessed. He said, "Of course, we all have our inconsistencies. Bill knows what he wants, which is a return on his investment, but when faced with the human condition, he will always try to make the right choice." This is the story I cherish most from my days as an advisor at the Gates Foundation.

One result of the decision to enter the fight against AIDS in January 2000 was that the Gates Foundation and Merck agreed to a joint program in Botswana to apply modern science under African conditions. Our first visit to Botswana was sobering. Over one-third of adults were HIV positive. The president of Botswana said that unless something dramatic was done they would no longer have a country.

AIDS was called a "radio disease" because while it was discussed on the radio, it was not discussed in ordinary conversation. Even at the increasing number of funerals, no mention was made of what everyone knew was the actual cause of death. The number of orphans was increasing. The impact on schools, medical facilities, and church programs was obvious. But discussion of the cause was muted. The only organization I encountered that would actually talk about AIDS openly was Hospice, a program resulting from the St. Christopher's Hospice, started by Dame Cicely Saunders in 1967, which inspired offshoots. This incredible organization has expanded around the world in the last two-thirds of a century and brings comfort to those dying and to their families.

We made rounds at a hospital in Botswana, and the reality hit home. Almost every patient had AIDS; yet, that diagnosis was never mentioned. Patients were said to have tuberculosis (which they did), cancer, and malnutrition but never AIDS.

At the completion of rounds, we went to a room to discuss what we had seen. I asked the medical officer, "How do you get yourself up in the morning? What do you do for your mental and emotional health?" He stared at me for such a long time that I regretted having asked the question and was seeking a way out. But then tears flowed down his face, and he said, "I have never told anyone this before." Then, in front of his staff and the visitors he said, "I was born one of four sons. My three brothers have died of AIDS. I don't have a choice."

The Gates Foundation, Merck, Harvard University, the government of Botswana, and others formed a coalition. Many things happened at once. Testing stations were developed so that people could know their HIV status. Treatment programs were established and quickly expanded. Being tested now made sense because a positive diagnosis would be followed by treatment. Education programs were launched, including a clever radio soap opera, sponsored by local actors and funded by USAID resources, that discussed AIDS frankly. Soon most people in the country were listening to the program and following the advice given.

A return to the country six years later revealed dramatic results. People were being tested and were receiving treatment. The shroud of secrecy had been lifted. On a visit to one of the testing facilities, I encountered a couple from the University of Botswana who had come for testing. They had agreed to be tested before becoming intimate. This type of discussion would have been beyond belief five years earlier.

Perhaps the most telling statistic comes from Luke Nkinsi. Dr. Nkinsi is an activist, a highly motivated African physician who has represented the Gates Foundation in the Botswana AIDS program. He reported that HIV positivity in newborns in Botswana had dropped from 40 percent when the program started to 4 percent within five years. These newborns can now develop, go to school, have careers, and raise families rather than exist only to occupy an early grave. Better health in Africa does not have to wait for development. It can become the engine of development.

chapter 25

BLIND SPOTS

Tradition is the DNA of our beliefs. The pull of tradition helps explain the strong emotions that accompany religious beliefs, political leanings, cultural values, and even food preferences.

In public health, one of the great challenges is to promote behavior change. We are all saddled with beliefs that make it hard to change, even in the face of great evidence. Tradition leads to many blind spots.

To reach a conclusion that was not held by my parents once seemed almost disrespectful. But then it became clear to me that they had raised us to think independently. My mother would reinforce this after a discussion on why we had reached a different conclusion, by saying, "You are never too old to learn from your children."

We all have blind spots. I am surprised at some of the things I believed even ten years ago, and I wonder how I could have been so blind. Likewise is the surprise of learning that large segments of the population can believe something long after it is proven untrue. Consider the evidence for global warming, which seems beyond the grasp of many in Congress, or the studies showing no relationship between vaccines and autism, which many refuse to accept. False beliefs in these two areas have a direct and negative impact on public health. But the mystery is larger.

Evolution

About half of the US population does not believe in evolution. Darwin was influenced by his religious grandfather, who used selective breeding to improve his domestic animals. This practice requires some understanding of evolution and the belief that it is possible to alter its course and speed. Every microbiologist sees evolution unfolding, sometimes within days. As mentioned earlier, the Westminster Dog Show is a convincing demonstration of evolution, as every breed exhibited has descended, through evolution, from wolves. Most scientists accept evolution as fact and proceed from there.

But half the population nevertheless believes that evolution is not compatible with religious beliefs and is therefore unable to take an open view of the evidence. There are plenty of ways to reconcile evolution with religious beliefs. Blind rejection is not one of them.

Women as Voters

Democracy holds leaders responsible to voters. This accountability is a powerful tool in causing political leaders to improve public health services, such as vaccines, safe water and food, clean air, and a safe environment. It becomes even more valuable if women also have the chance to vote and thereby influence public health decisions of political leaders. Mass delusion is yet another aspect of tradition, and so for almost a century and a half, the American tradition denied women the right to vote. There are still some who would argue that women should not be allowed to vote in this country. But their arguments do not carry the weight that they did 200 years ago. It is difficult for us to understand that once many men actually believed that their wives and mothers did not have the capacity to make an informed and intelligent choice in the voting booth but were able to make an informed and intelligent choice in choosing a husband.

But tradition is so strong that even when we concede the equality of women in voting, we continue our bias in the workplace. And, strangely, the belief that women are inferior continues in some Protestant and Catholic religious orders. To make it more mysterious, 50 percent of these church members, namely, the women, could leave churches that believe that they are not capable of being ministers or priests, but they do not leave. Do they actually believe the idea that they should not have the same rights as men? They do have the vote in the sense that they don't have to put up with it and yet they stay. Tradition.

Slavery

Throughout history, even in biblical stories, some people accepted the idea that some people should be able to enslave others. It is difficult to find Americans who will espouse that belief today. So how do we explain the lack of common sense that plagued large segments of the US population 160 years ago?

It cannot be explained by intelligence. Thomas Jefferson simply could not bring his intelligence to bear on his personal use of slaves. Likewise, in the 1840s, the president of Emory University led a committee that decided it was ethical for bishops to own slaves. Tradition often blocks rational thought.

Tradition was so strong that people were willing to die in large numbers to defend the irrational idea of slavery. They were willing to put civilians at risk, destroy homes and crops and families so that slavery would continue. They harmed the public's health. It defies our understanding today.

Tobacco

"And so it goes," as Kurt Vonnegut would say. While some had early suspicions that tobacco was a hazard to health, it took a surprisingly long time for the degree of that risk to be made clear. The degree of known risk now makes us think that it should have been crystal clear much sooner. But it was not. The early studies on the relationship of tobacco to lung cancer, for example, were weaker than expected because the control groups were often selected from hospitalized persons without lung cancer. Investigators were not aware that tobacco was also responsible for a large proportion of the other hospital admissions, such as heart disease, stroke, and other cancers; therefore, the strength of the relationship between tobacco and lung cancer was diluted by the fact that tobacco was so dangerous that it was also causing many of the problems in the control groups.

Gradually, it became clear that tobacco was toxic across the spectrum of disease problems. In a logical world, rapid action would have been taken to protect people from tobacco exposure to reduce the carnage. But the tobacco problem is made up of two parts—addiction and greed.

The addiction is intense. Solutions require helping those who would like to be freed as well as erecting barriers to make it more difficult for the young to become addicted. But greed stands in the way. The tobacco companies, to ensure their personal profit, came up with increasingly clever ways of getting young people simply *to try* smoking. Tobacco companies made smoking seem sophisticated; they sponsored concerts. They drew an association between smoking and manly pursuits, as seen in the Marlboro Man, or feminine ideals, as with Virginia Slims. Society looked the other way. Tobacco companies knew that, if they could get young people to smoke a single pack of cigarettes, many would be their slaves for the rest of their shortened lives.

The greed went beyond the tobacco executives and extended to the politicians who received donations from the tobacco companies, representatives of tobacco growers, or both. These same politicians intimidate public health experts who give testimony against tobacco products.

Even when the country was losing more than 1,000 lives a day to tobacco, tradition stifled a logical approach. One of every five funerals was the result of tobacco. In my speeches in the 1970s, I would say, "In other parts of our society, if someone makes their money by killing someone, we call that person a 'hit man.' Why don't we put the same label on tobacco executives, who know exactly how they are making their money?" Tradition is the answer.

In 2014, the problem remained. Smoking rates have decreased, and progress has been made, but how do we account for the fact that 400,000 Americans die each year because of tobacco? Why do public health departments continue to list the causes of death as heart disease, stroke, and cancer rather than saying the cause of death is tobacco? And how do we change a society that values greed over health? Newspapers should have a box score on the front page that keeps the tally on how many people died in that city in the past month because of tobacco. The *MMWR* could keep a tally on Americans lost so far this year because of tobacco, displayed in a box score on the front page of each issue.

Fifty years after the first *Surgeon General's Report* on tobacco, we continue to find the toll even higher than thought. In a hundred years, students will marvel at the collective blind spot involving tobacco, just as we now marvel over the blind spot this country had to slavery and as future generations will marvel at our blind spot to climate change.

Contraception

For some, viewing contraception as unacceptable is a tradition. It originated as a decision of humans, who then enveloped the idea in a cloak of infallibility. The evidence is that many ignore the idea that contraception is unacceptable, as shown by the low birth rates in traditional Catholic countries, such as Italy and France, and the similar rates of contraceptive use in Catholic versus non-Catholic families in the Americas. But poor families in poor countries have been slower to change their traditions. And meanwhile the population of the world has swollen, as have all of the problems resulting from excess population. The loss of rain forest in Africa, the acceleration of climate change, and the continuing problems of malnutrition, poverty, and the spread of infectious diseases, including Ebola, all result from the inability of many families to make logical decisions on family size and child spacing.

Counterintuitively, high infant death rates are compatible with the population explosion. It does not take much study to realize that the highest population growth rates are found in the countries with the highest infant and childhood death rates, while the lowest population growth rates are in the countries with the lowest infant and childhood death rates. Child health programs lead to improvements in family planning and contraception, which lead, in turn, to fewer infant deaths.

Gun Safety

There are many reasons for violence and the epidemic of gun deaths in the United States. Logical people would want to know as much about the problem as possible in order to offer solutions. But, in 1996, an amendment by Rep. Jay Dickey (R-Arkansas) withdrew funding from the CDC to study gun violence and threatened to withdraw all injury-control funds if the CDC included gun research as part of its mandate to do no harm. The NRA uses scare tactics about the government's having a long-term plan to take guns away from people. This is sufficient to make many act on the basis of fear rather than logic.

We look back in disbelief at the irrational actions of the past, only to realize that we continue to operate with misguided tradition, rather than with rational understanding of problems and solutions.

Medical Care

There will be a time when we will have to ask whether using the market-place was a good way to provide medical care in this country.

The facts are that the health indices of the United States—life expectancy, infant mortality, and chronic disease burdens—are not as good as in other industrialized countries. And these, after all, are the reasons for having a health care system. It is in place to reduce premature mortality and unnecessary suffering, not as a way to make money on illness. That should set off alarm bells that something is not working. We spend far more per person on health care than any other country and still cannot match their health outcomes. These facts should lead logical people to conclude that our system is not optimal.

Frequently, the response from politicians is, "We have the best health care system in the world, and we do not want to jeopardize it through socialized medicine." They are wrong. The United States does not even make it to the top twenty countries in the world when measuring health outcomes. It is an embarrassment to realize that about one-third of our health care expenditures do not go to health outcomes at all. They instead pay for the unneeded superstructure of insurance plans and managers that proliferate when profit, rather than quality and health outcomes, is the bottom line. Most of the twenty-plus countries with better health outcomes have single-payer systems. Our national response is that only the marketplace can improve health care delivery. If that is the case, why don't we prove it rather than just say it? A single-payer military system still allows for the use of marketplace forces to provide commodities and services. The United States continues to lead in expanding the science base of medicine. But it falls far behind other industrialized countries in improved health outcomes, coverage of the poor, and health equity.

Poverty

The current corollary to slavery is poverty. Poverty is very inconvenient to those in its grip, but it is also a burden to society. It is the single most important determinant of health. It is not just that poor people have poor health. Various studies have shown that the healthiest societies are those with the narrowest income inequality gap. Poverty breeds discontent, and the poor often attempt through crime or social disruption to remedy the disparities. Michael Manley, formerly the prime minister of Jamaica, once said that, "Poverty shared can be endured." Modern communications have demonstrated to the poor around the world that their condition is not being shared.

Six centuries ago, Emperor Hongzhi of China said that poverty should be seen in the same light as a person drowning or a person in a burning building. He said that in both these situations there is no time to lose, and the person must be rescued immediately.

No social determinant is as significant as poverty in causing poor health. It is not only the very poor who suffer reductions in health. Rather, every step down the income scale leads to an increase in health problems. Poverty, as a health problem, is dose related.

So poverty causes stigma and is a health hazard. But it is also similar to slavery in another regard: the poor actually subsidize the living standard for the rest of us. We get food, clothes, and lodging at a cheaper rate because people in this country and in other countries work at extremely low wages. In effect, we profit directly and indirectly from their poor standard of living in much the same way that plantation owners in the American South profited directly from the work of slaves. The embarrassment of the logic should be enough to lead to action even for those not interested in public health. But tradition salves the conscience of even the religious by repeating, "The poor will always be with us." That was a description of human foibles, not a law.

Public health workers need to focus on the effects of poverty but also on poverty itself. A living wage, rather than a minimum wage, needs to be established. No industry should be allowed to pay below that level. And the wage should be automatically indexed to inflation.

Fatalism

A close corollary to poverty, but separate in distribution, is fatalism. More common in the poor, but not restricted to them, this is the feeling that one cannot exert control over the future. It adversely affects health because it deters people from taking positive steps to improve health in the future. Fatalism is one of the reasons so many poor people continue to smoke in the face of information that shows the hazards. The poor often do not feel that they can control their future. But empowerment can be learned. The rich and the educated lost their fatalism as they saw what education and money could do to influence their future.

I emphasize to students that we are all a mixture of fatalism and empowerment and that the ratio changes with the day and the subject. It is important to believe that this is a cause-and-effect world, not a fatalistic one.

I am most fatalistic when I enter a taxi or an airplane. I have lost control. I often tell students of my experience in getting a taxi late at night at the Philadelphia airport. I suddenly was aware of the smell of alcohol. To judge the degree of risk, I engaged the driver in conversation. I said to him, "I need to tell you that I am a high-risk passenger." He asked, "What does that mean?" I told him that I had been involved in five taxi accidents in my lifetime, a true story. His reply was, "Oh that's nothing. I have been involved in a lot more than that."

chapter 26

ON BUDGETS AND BURGLARS

Real stories are often so much more interesting than the accepted accounts of how something happened. Polybius, several thousand years ago, said that the world is an organic whole, where everything interacts. This is a Polybius story.

The story began during my last year as director of the CDC. It was the last budget cycle for me as director. On Monday, I was to attend a meeting with Health and Human Services (HHS) secretary Richard Schweiker.

The budget process starts each year with the CDC's submitting, to the Public Health Service, the budget that the agency believes is required for the next year. The Public Health Service will inevitably remove some items entirely and reduce the request for other items in its attempt to balance the requests of all agencies. The Public Health Service then submits a budget for all of the agencies to HHS.

That department does its own review, usually removing more items, and almost never increasing a request. HHS then submits a consolidated budget to the White House. The White House (actually the Office of Management and Budget) makes decisions based on the entire federal government and sends its decisions back to the department. HHS then makes some changes, sending its conclusions to the Public Health Service. It, in turn, makes decisions, and the results are sent to the agencies, including the CDC. Every step up and down the line tends to remove requests that we felt were important when originally included. But we learned to accept the decisions.

However, one final opportunity existed to redress the most distressing reductions. This Monday meeting would be a chance, the last chance before the budget went to Congress, for the Public Health Service to make the agency's appeals to restore the program cuts that it found most appalling. It was an important meeting.

My family had spent the weekend out of town and returned home on Sunday night. I was well versed in the appeals that the CDC was seeking and therefore was not especially stressed in preparing for the meeting. I could do it with a few hours review that evening. But our calculations were immediately disrupted when we reached home that night. We had been burglarized. We called the police, and by the time they had left, and we had settled down, it was after midnight. I was up at 4:30 a.m. to get to the early-bird flight to Washington, DC. I was not feeling good because of sleep loss but also because of the violation inherent with a burglary.

A meeting was held first at the Public Health Service level to give us our marching orders. The instructions were a complete surprise. We were told that agency heads would not be allowed to speak, an approach I could not recall ever having been used in previous years. We were there only to answer questions if called on by the secretary. The budget professionals would handle the entire appeal process. My immediate thought was, *Why are we even here?*

Second, we were told that any attempt on our part to reinsert a capital project would result not only in the loss of that project but also in a loss of an equivalent amount of money from the remaining budget. This was hardball. The Reagan administration had decided that fiscal responsibility required no new building projects, no matter how important they were. This meant that our hopes for a Class-IV laboratory at the CDC would not be presented. I was informed of the three appeals the CDC would be allowed, but I had no input into the process.

We went to the secretary's meeting. NIH was the first agency reviewed. This is the largest agency in the Public Health Service, and, in truth, it is the best known and most watched by Congress. Any illness in congressional members, their families, or friends becomes a reason to provide an increase in appropriations. That is the reason much more money goes into research for cancer and heart disease than malaria, or other problems that involve far more people globally. The NIH appeal process went according to the rules. The director never said a word. *What a waste of his time,* I thought.

The CDC was next. Within the first minutes, the budget professionals got confused and could not figure out why they were having trouble reconciling two numbers. I sat on the sidelines and watched them try to stay in control. Secretary Schweiker listened for a few minutes and then with a bemused look said, "Bill is sitting right here. Couldn't we just ask him?" He then turned to me and said, "Why don't you present the CDC appeals?" It took me totally by surprise, but it was now out of the hands of the Public Health Service budget people.

I presented the first two appeals in a matter-of-fact way and then came to the third, and last, appeal. It concerned the immunization program. The White House had reduced the amount that we had requested. I believe that immunization is the foundation of public health. Vaccines allowed the modern era of public health to develop. Immunizations have a positive benefit-cost ratio, meaning that if you don't fund them, you have decided to continue having the problem but are spending more than prevention would have cost. It is an emotional issue with me. And I got emotional.

I told the secretary about the burglary. I told him that I still felt violated and upset when I got on the plane that morning but finally came to some accommodation with what had happened. I decided that the burglar knew I had more than he did and was trying to equalize the situation. But, I continued, as I looked at this last appeal, it brought back all of those feelings of having been violated, and it made me angry. The White House, I said, has now made a decision to "steal health from the American people. And no one seems to have the courage to stand up and say this is wrong."

The secretary turned to his budget officials and with no hesitation said, "Give him all three appeals." He then turned to me and asked, "Did you know it was going to be this easy?" I, of course, said no. He then asked, "If you had known it was going to be this easy, what would have been the fourth thing on your list?" The truth is that my fourth item would have actually been my first appeal, but we had been given firm instructions about not trying an end run on capital projects. However, I had never been offered an opportunity like this.

I looked at my boss, Ed Brandt, assistant secretary for health, and saw him put his head in his hands. He knew what I would ask for, and I had been ordered not to do that.

I went ahead. I told the secretary about Class-IV laboratories,* which deal with lethal agents for which we lack vaccines or treatment. I explained how the number of such agents had continued to increase and that the CDC

*Now known as BSL-4 laboratories.

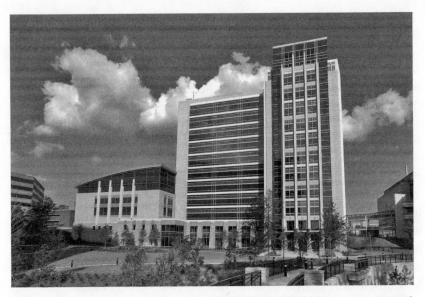

Emerging Infectious Diseases Laboratory, the CDC, 2005. This facility was constructed to triple the agency's capacity to conduct research and provide responses involving pathogens that require the highest levels of safety precautions. The Biosafety Lab-2 (BSL-2), BSL-3, and BSL-4 laboratory spaces provide the appropriate degree of containment for microorganisms under investigation. Photo from the CDC

had the capacity to deal with only one agent at a time. If a new suspicious agent came in, it meant closing down and cleaning the lab and then, after several days of effort, starting with the new unknown agent. The number of agents had increased but so had our diagnostic techniques. Everything was increasingly complicated, and we had our hands tied at the CDC.

The United States had only recently dealt with a problem of a person's putting poison in Tylenol bottles in drugstores. To make my case, I said to the secretary, "If we would be faced with a viral equivalent to the Tylenol problem, it would take less than an hour for the country to realize that we had no capacity to deal with it."

The secretary turned to his budget officers and said, "We have to at least try." It was about a week later when the secretary called me at home at night. He was calling from the White House, and he was as elated as a school-child. He told me that he had just gone head-to-head with David Stockman, director of the Office of Management and Budget.

"You will get your new lab," Secretary Schweiker said to me. He then told me that the administration was interested in speed; therefore, they were going to add it to the current year's budget so it would not even have to be

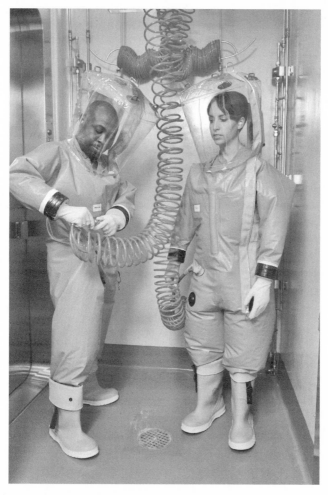

Inside a Class-IV laboratory at the CDC, 2007. Photo from the CDC

defended at the next congressional budget hearings. The secretary had understood the importance of this budget request. Suddenly, an important issue that appeared doomed a week earlier was on a fast track.

It is not an understatement to say that this lab has become absolutely essential to the CDC mission. Later, this became obvious when the CDC was dealing with Ebola virus, HIV, and West Nile viruses simultaneously.

Some years later, when I was executive director of the Carter Center, Jim Mason, the director of the CDC, invited me to attend the dedication of the new Class-IV laboratory building. It is a wonderful place, which provides for state-of-the-art diagnostic testing on multiple agents at one time.

It provides great flexibility in investigating our most serious and dangerous agents.

At the dedication, I heard, along with the rest of the audience, speeches about the logic behind the building and how it had come into being. And I thought to myself, *These people have no idea at all. We owe this building to two fumbling budget masters and an unknown Atlanta burglar.*

ACKNOWLEDGMENTS

The journey called writing a book would not be possible without many travel guides. I thank Ava Navin, a retired CDC editor, who donned a detective cap and scouted out elusive photographs and photographers. Aiding her and us in the photo hunt were Mary Hilpertshauser, historic collections manager at the David J. Sencer CDC Museum; Dennis Tolsma; Nancy Sterk; and Jim Curran.

Johns Hopkins University Press's staff have been patient, enthusiastic, and methodical in shepherding this publication. Special thanks to Robin W. Coleman, our acquisitions editor; Sahara Clement and Isla Hamilton-Short for managing the book's visuals; and Andre Barnett for her editing.

Finally, thank you to my anonymous reviewers for their time, attention, and many excellent suggestions to improve this book.

APPENDIX

Voices in My Head

We are the product of 1 million ancestors, since the Renaissance alone, and of countless associates who have encouraged us, helped us, worked beside us, and guided and nurtured us. Some are distinct voices in my head as I make decisions. Others, though they may be as important, are part of a chorus rather than soloists, so I may fail to point them out specifically.

To enlarge on each one of these mentors within this book might have been distracting, so here are more details on some of these voices in my head, for those who are interested. I know all but two of the people noted here—Jeanette Troup and Tommy Francis. I shared experiences with Jeanette, but never met her, and felt profoundly moved when she died of Lassa fever in Nigeria. Tommy Francis conducted a field study of inactivated polio vaccine so massive in its breadth and impact that I was moved to start a fund for students of global health, in his name, at the University of Washington.

This review highlights a major social change that continued after my departure from the CDC in 1984. Women were a distinct minority in medical and other scientific fields before that time. Female teachers in medical school were rare, and men constituted about 95 percent of the class. EIS officers at the CDC were usually men because the military draft did not include women. All of this changed during the second half of my career, which will greatly change the appendixes in my future books.

Personal Mentors

Of course, I will miss many as I start down this path but better to do that than miss the chance to mention any. This list is limited to those I knew personally, not those I knew only through their writings.

Family comes first: parents, brother, sisters, in-laws, and later my wife, Paula, and children, David, Michael, and Robert. I was later to learn how important my grandchildren, Max, Ella, Olyana, and Erika, can be in teaching and reteaching lessons on living.

Shirley and Jim Kohlstedt hired me at age 13 to work in their drugstore. They taught me, by example, how to treat people, the importance of passion in following professional pursuits or hobbies, and the necessity of meeting the public despite teenage shyness. (At this writing, Jim is in his 90s, and we continue to visit by phone.) Because of the Kohlstedts, I developed an interest in old cars, coin collecting, photography, and science.

Bill Strunk was a teacher of biology in college. He inspired fear in students and astonishment at the range and depth of his knowledge. He would begin lecturing before he entered the room and would go to the blackboard to write, using both hands simultaneously. I never got over my awe of him, but I became one of his lab assistants as well as a weekend gardener at his home. His bluster hid a kind and helpful core that provided support for my admission to medical school.

Medical school was exciting and demanding, but few faculty members had an interest in global health. The exception was Rei Ravenholt, Seattle King County epidemiologist and teacher in the medical school. He employed me after school and on weekends and shared his passions for many things. He advised me that, if I was interested in global health, I should seek entrance into the EIS. His letter of recommendation was crucial in my reaching that goal. (At this writing, he is in his 90s, and we continue to communicate by phone and periodic lunches.)

Alex Langmuir, the creator of the EIS, is a legend. He was feared by many but a supporter and advocate for those working for him. He taught respect for numbers and the need for rigor in interpreting them. He had incredible confidence in his abilities and the power of epidemiology and passed that confidence on to those working for him.

Tom Weller became my mentor by chance. Reading a commencement address he had given at the Harvard Medical School, published in the *New England Journal of Medicine*, I was struck by his ability to put into words concepts that I believed but had never seen written so clearly in regard to global health. He wrote about equity and the skills and knowledge we possess but don't share in full measure with the parts of the world in great need of them. (See chapter 8.) I applied to spend a year studying with him, only then learning he was a Nobel laureate. We forged a bond that lasted until his death at age 93.

Charlie Houston, cardiologist, mountain climber, high-altitude physiologist, and professor, also came into my life by chance, when I volunteered as a Peace Corps physician in India in 1962. Charlie became an important contributor to my life philosophy. He was an icon in the climbing community, worked on the development of an artificial heart, continued high-altitude physiology work all of his life, and provided a daily example of tenacity in the most difficult situations, all without complaining. Again, I developed a lifetime bond with him and had an exhilarating phone conversation with him weeks before he died at age 96. (I have been fortunate to have long-term connections with my mentors—but also many have thrived into old age.)

Frank Neva was my faculty advisor at Harvard. He was successful in three fields—research, teaching, and clinical medicine—simultaneously, a rarity. He was generous in his time as an advisor and a pleasure to converse with throughout his life until his death at age 89. His son-in-law, Peter Bell, was involved in my selection to direct the CDC in 1977.

Wolfgang Bulle was a surgeon educated in Germany during World War II. He was a gifted physician, who spent his life seeking redemption for his country's role in that war. He could never work hard enough to ease his mind. I was grateful for his support in my work in Africa and for his continuing support when the CDC hired me to work on smallpox eradication. He provided an extreme example of tenacity.

Yemi Ademola headed preventive medicine in Nigeria. He came from a famous Yoruba family. Yemi was an example of compassion, competence, and absolute integrity. I met him as a classmate during the year I spent with Tom Weller at Harvard. Yemi became president of our class. In our yearbook, he wrote that no field of knowledge lies outside the interest of public health professionals. He was helpful in Paula's and my early work with a medical center in Eastern Nigeria and with the launching of the Smallpox Eradication/Measles Control Program in Nigeria. With years of service still to be donated to his country, he was murdered by an intruder in his home a few years after graduation. The feeling of loss continues almost fifty years later.

Adetokunbo Lucas had just graduated from the Harvard School of Public Health in 1964 when I met him at the CDC. He provided an important intervention during a tense meeting in Lagos in 1967, crucial in my ability to pursue surveillance/containment strategies for the elimination of smallpox. We interacted constantly through the years as he worked at the WHO, Harvard, and Carnegie Corporation, including visits he made to the Carter Center and the Gates Foundation. Our friendship continues in his 84th year.

David Sencer directed the CDC for eleven years and was both a supervisor and a friend during that time and the years after. As a mentor, he both taught and caused concern. The teaching involved his ability to know everything, to prowl the halls of the CDC, dropping in to see people and to ask them to explain what they were doing. He had the pulse of the organization and was supportive and interested. The concern came from those same qualities; that is, he knew everything and had the kind of mind that could instinctively extract the relevant pieces of information important to the matter at hand. (I think it may be near impossible to *learn* this skill.) He invested domestic resources globally to eradicate smallpox, arguing that was the correct way to protect Americans. And his strategies fulfilled the demands of Congress that such global investments be shown to help Americans: the United States recoups its investment in smallpox eradication every three months.

Bill Watson, deputy director of the CDC during my time as director, was a superb manager, who combined great skills in finding ways to achieve objectives but always with the highest degree of integrity. He was a mentor not only for me but for everyone at the CDC. He also had an insatiable desire for knowledge and took a keen interest in politics. The day could not legally start at work until a discussion on current events was concluded. Few people have influenced me so continuously in work, had his understanding of the total environment in which we work, or had his ability to stay focused on outcomes.

As with Bill Watson, Stu Kingma—who was a unique combination of an intellectual, skilled craftsman, and philosopher—was a product of the group of investigators for the program on sexually transmitted diseases. The best of these public health advisors became great managers for other CDC programs. Stu was in that category. He was obsessive about doing the best job possible, but he was also philosophical and thoughtful. His answers to questions were always thought through. He worked in a variety of CDC programs, including smallpox eradication in India. We share a friendship in our ninth decade of life.

Stan Foster has been a friend and mentor since we shared our first days at the CDC in July 1962. We both worked in the EIS, on smallpox eradication in Nigeria, and on smallpox in Asia. We both had careers at the CDC and then both joined the faculty at the Rollins School of Public Health at Emory University. Stan worked in some of the most difficult places in the smallpox days and became a mentor not only for me but for countless students in other countries and at Emory.

Don Millar was the person who called me to say I had been accepted into the EIS. We switched roles at various times, as he supervised me and later I supervised him. He was bright, aggressive, and always a leader who could get things done. I learned from him for half a century.

M. I. D. Sharma was one of the calmest managers under pressure that I have seen. He was in charge of malaria eradication in India at one time but was in charge of smallpox eradication when I met him. He was wise in the way he handled people. He did not intimidate them so much as he made them want to serve him well. His stellar reputation made him a leader and a mentor for many of us.

P. Diesh, a gruff, experienced career medical officer, who answered to the minister of health of India, was initially an enigma to me. I was put off by his apparent low regard for women or workers under his supervision. It was some time before I realized his approach was based on a fear of not being respected if he did not display power. In truth, he was very concerned about those under him and became increasingly comfortable in dealing with women. And he was so effective. Give him any problem and he would pick up the phone and badger someone until the problem was solved. Nothing stood in his way. In retirement, he told me how meaningful smallpox eradication had become for him and that he would come out of retirement if we could find another such challenge.

Mahendra Dutta, another career medical officer in the upper echelons of India's Ministry of Health, was similar to Sharma in his calm approach to disastrous problems. He was unafraid to express opinions, even to a minister of health. The second of a three-generation public health family, inspired by a Rockefeller Foundation fellowship to his father in the 1940s, he traveled constantly to the field. With his measured tones, he was able to get work out of everyone. Forty-one years after the last case of smallpox in India, we continue to communicate and be friends.

Jacob John received his medical training in the United States and turned down many offers to stay in this country. He returned to India to become head of pediatrics at Vellore Medical School. His scientific acumen, research abilities, clear thinking, writing, and speaking—plus his extraordinary compassion—have made him an important mentor for decades.

Nicole Grasset was in a league of her own. A fearless physician who drove alone from Delhi to Paris at the completion of smallpox eradication in Southeast Asia, she accepted no bureaucratic obstacles. She once wrote a letter to Prime Minister Indira Gandhi when she was unable to get the system to respond to her requests. She mixed scientific abilities with compassion, graciousness, and fashion to become an example to all.

Julius Richmond took pediatric training before World War II and became a flight surgeon during the war. He made his mark in medicine, eventually becoming surgeon general of the United States. But his interests were broad, and he cofounded the Head Start program. He was tireless in his pursuit of better health for everyone until his death at age 92.

Ed Brandt combined medicine, a degree in biostatistics, and a background in theology to become the assistant secretary of health in the Reagan administration. He was as solid in that position as anyone could be. Low key but intense and always learning, he welcomed advice, rewarded good ideas, and brought an ethical framework to his decisions.

Everett Koop, a pediatric surgeon, became surgeon general with the backing of the religious right. He continued to surprise his base by looking at the science, supporting abortion surveillance programs, and speaking out on the need for humane responses to the AIDS epidemic. He was a delight to work with and became an important health symbol in conveying information to the public.

Richard Schweiker went from senator in Pennsylvania to the secretary of Health and Human Services under President Reagan. He was very able and would give proper attention to scientific evidence. He was comfortable in asking agencies for information when layers of government obscured the message. His interest in global health was an important signal and demonstrated his ability to provide leadership in difficult times.

So many political leaders provided leadership to the CDC. Senator Mark Hatfield was interested in global health and in making sure that the CDC was getting proper budgetary attention. Senator Paul Simon traveled to Africa and was interested in health and education on that continent. He was a strong supporter of nutrition programs in low-income countries and always voted his conscience. Senator Edward Kennedy not only took public health seriously but also would call frequent hearings to be sure the CDC was being heard. He even held a hearing on Legionnaires' disease at the CDC in Atlanta. Congressman Henry Waxman never missed an opportunity to promote public health. Congressman Paul Rogers was one of the kindest people in Congress. He was always fair to witnesses, and his courtesy was legendary. At his memorial service, one person asked for a show of hands from anyone who had ever followed him through a door. Not a hand went up because he always insisted on the other person going first. Congressman Bill Lehman provided money for three years to expand the

CDC program on injury control. Finally, he could not be ignored by the Department of Health and Human Services, and it included the money directly into the CDC budget.

I need to mention the only man who was so interested in health that he asked for a private tutorial. Senator Bob Graham from Florida was so committed to improving his health legislative skills that he asked us to arrange a tutorial for him. We planned for a series of the top people from various branches of medicine to instruct him, and he set aside an hour a week, over a period of many months, for the project.

Colleagues

Even more numerous than mentors are the many colleagues, in and out of the workplace, who helped in achieving health objectives. Their influence goes far beyond any stories in this book.

Connie and Lyle Conrad, both physicians, were in the Peace Corps in Nigeria before their time at the Harvard School of Public Health. Lyle went on to head the program for EIS field staff at the CDC. He spent long hours on the phone providing guidance, always taking copious notes. He was in an ideal position to suggest people for short-term work in smallpox eradication and disaster relief. Connie went on to head a program at Emory University. It started as a master's program in community health and then grew to a master's in public health. Eventually, Emory developed a school of public health, now in the top half-dozen schools in the country.

Jeanette Troup, known to me only by reputation as mentioned earlier, was the only doctor at the Jos, Nigeria, hospital that admitted the first known Lassa fever patient. She was well trained and exceedingly well liked by the staff and patients at the hospital. Coworkers described her singing as professional, and indeed she often entertained the staff with music. After medical school, she took residencies in both pediatrics and pathology so she was well equipped to do an autopsy on a Lassa fever patient in 1970. And yet she slipped, cut her finger, and died of Lassa fever. Her tragic story is told in the book *Fever: The Hunt for a New Killer Virus,* by John G. Fuller.

Karl Johnson was head of the Special Pathogens Laboratory at the CDC, investigating the most deadly viral diseases. While highly regarded for his calm ability to confront hemorrhagic viral diseases, he describes himself as being absolutely scared in dealing with the first known Ebola outbreak in Zaire in 1976. Until he was convinced the virus was not spreading through the air, he said the investigators could not relax. In retirement, he continues to respond to many requests for consultation.

Joel Breman was a veteran of the smallpox program in West Africa. He was also part of the initial team to investigate Ebola in Zaire in 1976. He continued his career in global health at the National Institutes of Health and served on assessment teams to verify that smallpox had truly disappeared from the world. He is doing comparable work on verifying the elimination of Guinea worm.

Joe McCormick also became a career global health worker. He originally went to Zaire as a science teacher, became interested in medicine, and returned to the United States to go to medical school. He became interested in virology and participated in the first Ebola outbreaks. He later went to Sierra Leone to study Lassa fever and was able to determine its epidemiology from rodents to people and worked on approaches to treatment.

Peter Piot worked on the original Zaire Ebola outbreak before becoming deeply immersed in the problem of AIDS in the 1980s. He was named the first director of the Joint United Nations Programme on HIV and AIDS (UNAIDS), traveling around the world to secure resources and to help countries develop national programs. He is now the dean of the London School of Tropical Medicine.

Don Francis, in a career devoted to global health problems, has worked in Africa, South America, and Asia. He joined a WHO team to control an Ebola outbreak in southern Sudan, one that actually preceded the first recognized outbreak of that disease, in Zaire in 1976. The outbreaks were found to be caused by slightly different strains. Don went on to work on smallpox eradication in India and Bangladesh. He later conducted the first human trials with an AIDS vaccine in Thailand and the United States.

David Fraser's work with Legionnaires' disease is recounted in this book. Fraser went on to have a varied career, which included the presidency of Swarthmore from 1982 to 1991. At that time, he left to become the head of the Social Welfare Department at the Aga Khan Secretariat, where he directed health, education, and housing activities in Asia and Africa. Moreover, he has been named by the Pennsylvania Guild of Craftsmen as a Master Artisan, using ancient arts to make contemporary baskets.

Mark Rosenberg worked in enteric diseases as an EIS officer and spent time in India for smallpox eradication. He started the program on injury control at the CDC, work that was highly praised and included state health department programs and academic centers for injury control research. Mark went on to great success at the Task Force for Global Health, including serving as director for seventeen years. That group focuses on neglected diseases in poor countries.

Joseph McDade described himself as a "back bencher," out of the limelight in a small lab at the CDC, at the time of the Legionnaires' disease outbreak. His lab was asked to rule out Q fever in that investigation. This infection with *Coxiella burnetii,* a bacterium, didn't really fit the clinical pattern being seen with Legionnaires' disease, as it causes a flulike illness that can progress to atypical pneumonia. Nonetheless, the CDC's plan was to exclude any infectious disease known to science. Six months after the outbreak, Joe McDade discovered the problem, both because he was compulsive and returned to the lab between Christmas and New Year's to sort through the past year, but also because he was disturbed by a man at a holiday party who said that he expected better of the CDC. Joe repeated the process originally used to rule out Q fever and found a small clue that led to the unraveling of the mystery of Legionnaires' disease.

Charlie Shepard was chief of the Leprosy and Rickettsia Branch at the CDC for more than thirty years. He had a reputation for being a superb scientist, who advanced the understanding of leprosy. At one time, that organism could not be grown in the laboratory. Shepard pioneered ways of growing it in the footpads of mice. Later he worked with the nine-banded armadillo, which provided abundant opportunities for growing and studying leprosy. He supervised Joe McDade, and he helped to isolate *Legionella* organisms (chapter 9). He was approachable and acted as a mentor for many CDC scientists.

Walter Dowdle was another revered scientist at the CDC. He had wide and varied experiences with laboratory techniques but especially concentrated on the baffling role of the influenza virus as it mutated to essentially become a new threat every few years. His wide-ranging interests and leadership abilities led him to head the Center for Infectious Diseases at the CDC in 1977. He later became deputy director of the CDC and provided oversight for the *Morbidity and Mortality Weekly Report* (*MMWR*). On his retirement from the CDC in 1994, he became involved in polio eradication and helped to establish diagnostic laboratories around the world to support that effort.

Don Berreth directed the Office of Public Affairs at the CDC. Raised in South Dakota, he spent five years as a press officer for the FDA. He spent the rest of his career at the CDC. He had exceptional judgment and was called on repeatedly to advise on developments both within and outside of the CDC. He was trusted by journalists and had a reputation for making the people working on a particular problem available to the press, rather than using the Office of Public Affairs as a filter. He died at age 57 of a virulent staphylococcal infection.

Gene Matthews spent twenty-five years as the CDC's counsel. He was also an advisor on many situations beyond his immediate responsibility and a leader in using the law to improve the health of the public. In his early years, he served as attorney-advisor to the Micronesian Claims Commission, stationed in the Mariana Islands. On retirement from the CDC, he went to the North Carolina School of Public Health and has concentrated on making the law a potent tool to improve health throughout the world.

David Thompson worked on smallpox eradication in Eastern Nigeria during the first year of that program. He later became a missionary in Chad and had great success in developing village health programs that were staffed by local workers provided with basic training to treat the most common conditions they encountered. He was part of the global health successes in transferring skills and knowledge to poor areas of the world.

Mike Lane played a major role in the eradication of smallpox with oversight responsibilities for many countries in the CDC's West Africa program. He played a leading role in determining the risks of smallpox vaccine and in ending the use of that vaccine in the United States even before smallpox was eradicated from the rest of the world. He taught public health at the University of California, Berkeley, and at the Emory University Rollins School of Public Health.

Don Hopkins is a gifted pediatrician and global health worker, who demonstrated the surveillance/containment smallpox strategy in Sierra Leone. He headed the CDC global health efforts before joining the Carter Center, where he became the director of health activities and the major force behind Guinea worm eradication. He documented the history of smallpox in a popular book, *The Greatest Killer: Smallpox in History*, and is doing the same for Guinea worm.

George Lythcott was a pediatrician working in Ghana on pulmonary disease research when the CDC hired him to head up the new regional office in Lagos for smallpox eradication and measles control. He was an intuitive politician, who could negotiate easily with African governments. The same skills were useful when he later served as a dean at the City University Medical School in New York, as associate dean at Columbia University, associate vice chancellor at the University of Wisconsin, and administrator of the Health Services Administration for the Department of Health and Human Services. I was in awe of his ability to talk himself out of any dilemma we encountered during our many years of working together.

Rafe Henderson combined a strong academic background in medicine and public health plus a degree from the Kennedy School at Harvard, with communication skills in both English and French that allowed for superb leadership first in smallpox eradication and later as head of the WHO program to expand childhood immunizations to all children. He was able to persuade others to share his vision and then methodically plan strategies to achieve that vision. He continues to inspire.

Don Eddins was a Texan with a soft approach. He was able to develop statistical techniques and polling approaches useful to programs working in poor areas of the world that lacked addresses or census information. He was methodical and prized order in his approach to record keeping and distribution of information.

Seth Leibler brought a refreshing approach to training at the CDC. He had been trained in criterion-referenced instruction, in which training is graded by previously determined criteria that indicate success. The approach was highly relevant to the CDC, and this concept was taken to ongoing tasks, such as how to provide a system for responding to a smallpox importation into this country. He developed his own consulting firm to teach his approach to business clients.

Olen Kew is a virologist with a PhD from the University of Washington and a creative mind, put to good use in combatting the frustrating disease of polio. Polio can infect hundreds of people before the first clinical signs are apparent in a person with muscle weakness. It has been known since 1962 that oral polio vaccine can revert to a dangerous virus that can circulate and cause polio disease.

Kew has been involved in tracing such reversions and is in the forefront of developing scientific tests and approaches to eliminate polio from the world.

Tommy Francis was the first scientist to isolate influenza virus. He became the mentor to many virologists, including Jonas Salk. It was Francis who convinced Salk that a field trial was needed for his new inactivated polio vaccine. Francis then ran a study of 1.8 million children, plus hundreds of thousands of volunteers, to determine the efficacy of the vaccine. It is because paralysis is so rare with polio—only a single case may occur in hundreds of children with the disease—that the study had to be so large. The study was completed in less than two years, before the advent of computers, and is the largest field study ever undertaken in the field of vaccines. His son-in-law, Russ Alexander, was a teacher of mine in medical school, and his daughter became a minister. They were both retired in Seattle at the time of the fiftieth anniversary of the Francis field trial.

Paul Wiesner is mentioned for his role in beginning the first CDC investigation of AIDS. He was head of the venereal disease program at that time. Paul also went on to head the DeKalb County Board of Health, where he was honored for providing extraordinary leadership. He was president of the National Association of County and City Health Officials (NACCHO), a group numbering about 3,000 health leaders. Paul is a solid scientist and mentor to many.

Alan Hinman has fifty years of involvement in global health. He directed the Immunization Division at the CDC during the expansion of that program to cover all children in the United States. He retired from the CDC in 1996 and continued to work in global immunization programs with the Task Force for Global Health. He still provides global leadership, especially in the areas of polio and measles eradication.

Walter Orenstein had intended to become a pediatric nephrologist. A field assignment in India for smallpox eradication became a life-changing event for him, however, and he returned to the CDC to devote his life to vaccine-preventable diseases. He headed the national program when the United States hit the lowest level of vaccine-preventable diseases in history. He played a major role in advising other countries and the WHO on their immunization activities. He now works at Emory University on the continuing improvement of vaccine programs for the world.

Joan Davenport was the nerve center for the early smallpox program in West and Central Africa. She not only supported the Atlanta headquarters but also became the go-to person for those in the field. She was unflappable, organized, and cheerful, making a host of new incoming workers comfortable at the CDC.

Carol Walters, my assistant at the CDC and later a cofounder of the Task Force for Child Survival, spent many years in global health activities. Well-organized, perceptive, and friendly, she provided a welcoming environment to the many visitors seeking advice. She demonstrated the role of good management in making programs work and was able to reduce the stress level of those of us working in her team.

Anne Mather has her master's degree in journalism and spent years as the managing editor of the *MMWR* at the CDC. She is the author or coauthor of ten books, most recently one with Mary Guinan, *Adventures of a Female Medical Detective: In Pursuit of Smallpox and AIDS*, on Guinan's career as an epidemiologist. Anne has been involved for years in rug hooking and has published books on that craft, advising hookers (that is indeed what they call themselves) to infuse their personality into the rugs they create. She has made writing accessible for me, saved me from many bad ideas, and made the process fun.

And More to Come . . .

I was to have even more mentors as I aged. A subsequent book will pay tribute to Jim Curran, Norman Borlaug, President Jimmy Carter and Mrs. Rosalynn Carter, Jim Laney (president of Emory University), Melinda Gates, Bill Gates Sr., Bill Gates Jr., and Patty Stonesifer.

REFERENCES

Chapter 3
1. CDC. Lassa [Video documentary]. Atlanta, GA: CDC; 1998.
2. Von Drehle D. The ones who answered the call. Time. Dec. 22, 2014. pp. 70–107.

Chapter 4
1. Reid RW. Microbes and men. New York: Saturday Review Press; 1975.
2. Holmes OW. The contagiousness of puerperal fever. New England Quarterly Journal of Medical Surgery. 1843;1503-30.
3. Loudon I. Alexander Gordon and puerperal fever. ACP News. 2003 Autumn. pp. 26-38.
4. Jenner E. An inquiry into the causes and effects of the variolae vaccinae, or cow-pox. 1798. Published in The Harvard Classics; 1909-14.
5. Jones B. Joe Mountin Lecture. 4th Annual Mountin Lecture, Oct. 26, 1983. CDC, Atlanta.
6. Watson J. The double helix: A personal account of the discovery of the structure of DNA. New York: Atheneum; 1968.

Chapter 5
1. Ravenholt RT, Foege WH. Epidemiology and treatment of lung cancer in Seattle. Diseases of the Chest. 1963;44:174-85.
2. Foege WH. House on fire: The fight to eradicate smallpox. Berkeley: University of California Press; 2011.
3. Foege WH, Leland OS, Mollohan CS, Fulginiti VA, Henderson DA, Kempe CH. Inactivated measles-virus vaccine. Public Health Reports. 1965;80:60-64.

Chapter 7
1. CDC. Toxic-shock syndrome—United States. MMWR. 1980;29(25):229-30.

Chapter 8
1. Schweitzer A. Out of my life and thought. New York: Henry Holt; 1933. Republished by Baltimore: Johns Hopkins University Press; 1998.
2. Weller TH. Questions of priority. New England Journal of Medicine. 1963;269(13):673-78.

Chapter 10
1. Foege WH. House on fire: The fight to eradicate smallpox. Berkeley: University of California Press; 2011.

Chapter 14

1. McGinnis JM, Foege WH. Actual causes of death in the United States. Journal of the American Medical Association. 1993;270(18):2207-12.
2. Idler EL, editor. Religion as a social determinant of public health. London: Oxford University Press; 2014.
3. Donne J. Meditation XVII. 1624.
4. Einstein A. Speech at the California Institute of Technology. As quoted in New York Times. Feb. 16, 1931.

Chapter 15

1. Offit PA. The Cutter incident. New Haven: Yale University Press; 2005.
2. Nader R. Scientists or celebrities? CounterPunch. Apr. 16, 2005.
3. Protecting the world's children: Vaccines and immunization within primary health care. A Bellagio Conference. Mar. 13-14, 1984. Rockefeller Foundation, New York.
4. Deer B. How the case against the MMR vaccine was fixed. British Medical Journal. 2011;342:c5347.
5. Godlee F, Smith J, Marcovitch H. Wakefield's article linking MMR vaccine and autism was fraudulent [Editorial]. British Medical Journal. 2011;342:c7452.

Chapter 16

1. Kohn LT, Corrigan JM, Donaldson MS (Institute of Medicine). To err is human: Building a safer health system. Washington, DC: National Academies Press; 2000.
2. Foege WH. Budgetary medical ethics [Guest editorial]. Journal of Public Health Policy. 1981;2(1):8-18.
3. Linn R, Stuart SL. The last chance diet: When everything else has failed; Dr. Linn's protein-sparing fast program. Secaucus, NJ: Lyle Stuart; 1976.

Chapter 17

1. Fleck F. Consensus during the Cold War: Back to Alma-Ata. Bulletin of the World Health Organization. 2008;86(10):745-46.

Chapter 19

1. Zimbardo P. The Lucifer effect: Understanding how good people turn evil. New York: Random House; 2007.

Chapter 20

1. Reye RDK, Morgan G, Baral J. Encephalopathy and fatty degeneration of the viscera: A disease entity in childhood. Lancet. 1963;282(7311):749-52.
2. Johnson GM, Scurletis TD, Carroll NB. A study of sixteen fatal cases of encephalitis-like disease in North Carolina children. North Carolina Medical Journal. 1963;24:464-73.
3. Starko KM, Ray CG, Dominguez LB, Stromberg WL, Woodall DF. Reye's syndrome and salicylate use. Pediatrics. 1980;66(6):859-64.
4. CDC. Follow-up on Reye syndrome—United States. Epidemiologic Notes and Reports. MMWR. 1980;29:321-22.
5. CDC. Reye syndrome—Ohio, Michigan. MMWR. Reprinted from Nov. 7, 1980, as a landmark article in 1997;46(32):750-55.

6. CDC. National surveillance for Reye syndrome, 1981: Update, Reye syndrome and salicylate usage. MMWR. 1982;31:53-56.
7. CDC. Surgeon General's advisory on the use of salicylates and Reye syndrome. MMWR. 1982;31(22):289-90.
8. Committee on Infectious Diseases, American Academy of Pediatrics. Aspirin and Reye syndrome [Special report]. Pediatrics. 1982;69(6):810-12.
9. CDC. Reye syndrome—United States, 1984. MMWR. 1985;34(1):13-16.
10. CDC. Reye syndrome—United States, 1985. MMWR. 1986;35(5):66-68, 73-74.

Chapter 21

1. Singh M. Cosmic reflections of health for all. Ottawa, Ontario: Le Cercle des Amis de Mohan Singh; 1983.
2. Singh M. Maxims II, son of cosmic reflections. Ottawa, Ontario: Le Cercle des Amis de Mohan Singh; 1988.
3. de Leeuw E. The boulder in the stream. Health Promotion International. Dec. 2011;26(Suppl. 2):ii157-60.
4. Ayres JC. Decelerating skyrocketing health-care cost. New England Journal of Medicine. 1977;296(7):391-93.
5. Singh M. Letters to the editor. New England Journal of Medicine. 1977;296:1540.

Chapter 22

1. Institute of Medicine. Injury in America: A continuing public health problem. Washington, DC: National Academies Press; 1985.

Chapter 24

1. CDC. *Pneumocystis* pneumonia—Los Angeles. MMWR. 1981;30(21):250-52.
2. CDC. A cluster of Kaposi's sarcoma and *Pneumocystis carinii.* MMWR. 1982;31(23):305-7.
3. Jaffe HW, Choi K, Thomas PA, Haverkos HW, Auerbach DM, Guinan ME, Rogers MF, et al. National case-control study of Kaposi's sarcoma and *Pneumocystis carinii* pneumonia in homosexual men: Part 1. Epidemiologic results. Annals of Internal Medicine. 1983;99(2):145-51.
4. Auerbach DM, Darrow WW, Jaffe HW, Curran JW. Cluster of cases of the acquired immune deficiency syndrome: Patients linked by sexual contact. American Journal of Medicine. 1984;76:487-92.
5. CDC. *Pneumocystis carinii* pneumonia among persons with hemophilia A. MMWR. 1982;31:365-67.
6. CDC. Prevention of acquired immune deficiency syndrome (AIDS): Report of interagency recommendations. MMWR. 1983;32:101-3.
7. Barre-Sinoussi F, Chermann JC, Rey F, et al. Isolation of a T-lymphotropic retrovirus from a patient at risk for acquired immune deficiency syndrome (AIDS). Science. 1983;220(4599):868-71.
8. Gallo RC, Salahuddin SZ, Popovic M, et al. Frequent detection and isolation of cytopathic retroviruses (HTLV-III) from patients with AIDS and at risk for AIDS. Science. 1984;224:500-503.

INDEX

Page locators in italics signify photos.

Ademola, Yemi, 52-53, 106, 243
Advisory Committee on Immunization Practices, 59, 95, 146
AID Atlanta, 219
AIDS, 209-24; in Africa, 213-14, 217-18, 221-24; antiviral drugs for, 219-20; and blood supply, 214-15; and George W. Bush administration, 161, 220; CDC response to, 27, 154, 172-73, 210-15; discovery of virus causing, 215-17; and gay community, 219; in Haiti, 214; and hemophiliacs, 212-13, 214; Kaposi's sarcoma in, 210-11
Alexander, Russ, 34, 250
Allen, Ivan, Jr., 114
American Academy of Pediatrics, 146
American Journal of Medicine, 212
American Medical Association, 168, 184
Amish, 134-35
Anderson, Jack, 65
Annals of Internal Medicine, 211-12
antibiotics, 83, 105, 126, 152, 168
anticancer vaccines, 138, 147
Arnold of Villanova, 108-9
autism, 144-46, 225
Averroes, 109
Azu, Charles, 52

Bacon, Francis, 109
Bacon, Roger, 109
Bangladesh, 187, 188; cyclone in, 90-91
Baral, J., 179-80
Barré-Sinoussi, Françoise, 216
Bartter syndrome, 43-44
BCG (Bacille Calmette Guerin) vaccine, 53
Bell, Peter, 207, 242
Bellamy, Carol, 142
Berkley, Seth, 143, 217, 218
Berreth, Don, 67, 103, 123, 248
Biafra, 72, 73, 79, 86
Biden, Joe, 199

Bill & Melinda Gates Foundation, 143, 218-19, 221, 222-24, 251
bioterrorism, 1-3, 31
bloodletting, 20
Botswana, 223-24
botulinum toxin, 1-2
Bourne, Peter, 155
Boutwell, Joseph, 65
Brandling-Bennett, David, 159
Brandt, Ed, 173, 183, 216, 235; and NIOSH, 176, 177; portrayal of, 205, 245
Breman, Joel, 11, 12, 246-47
British Medical Journal, 145-46
Buchwald, Art, 205-7, *206*
Buckley, Sonja, 8
Bulle, Gisela, 90
Bulle, Wolfgang, 54-55, 80, 90, 148, 242-43
Bulletin of the World Health Organization, 157
Bumpers, Dale and Betty, 135, 171
Bush, George W., 160, 161, 220

Califano, Joseph, 100-101, 102-3, 135, 174, 202-3
Canada, 158-59
Cantor, Eddie, 131
Carter, Jimmy, 45, 100, 135, 150, 204, 207, 208, 218, 251
Carter, Rosalynn, 135, *165,* 208, 251; visit to refugee camps by, 162, 163, 164-65, 166
Carter Center, 219, 237, 249
Casals, Jordi, 8
Center for Environmental Health, 175-76
Center for Infectious Diseases, 111-12
Center for Injury Control, 198
Centers for Disease Control (CDC): and AIDS crisis, 27, 172-73, 209-15; and Bartter syndrome, 43-46; bioterrorism strategy of, 2-3; Birth Defects Branch of, 43; BSL-4 laboratories, 235-38, *236, 237*; CASE program of, 95-96; and Congress, 48, 64-66, 150-51, 170-78, 199, 245-46; and Cutter incident, 117, 133-34; daily

Centers for Disease Control (CDC) (*cont.*) operations of, 116-18; and Ebola outbreak, 11, 12-13, 16; and EIS officers, 30-32, 113, 124, 86-90; and Emory University, 24-25, 27; epidemiology as emphasis of, 22, 28, 107; equal employment opportunities at, 114-16; Foege selection as director of, 101-3; formation of, 21, 22, 23; funding of, 111, 167, 199, 233-38; global health concerns of, 30, 86-90, 153-56, 159-60; health risk appraisals by, 5-6; humor at, 187-94; immunization programs of, 120-21, 135-38; as information provider, 120; and injury control, 195-99, 247; international visitors to, 155-58; and Lassa fever outbreak, 7-10; and last polio outbreak, 134-35; and Legionnaires' disease, 62-68; and *MMWR,* 119-20; NIOSH division of, 175-78; partnerships for, 119-20; public health as mission of, 30, 104, 105-6, 120-21; relations with state and local agencies, 40-41, 124; reorganization of, 111-12; and Reye syndrome, 181-86; security at, 4-6; smallpox eradication efforts of, 5, 13, 36-38, 70-78, 83, 91, 93, 96-97, 153, 154; structure of, 106-7; and swine flu epidemic, 49, 58-63; and toxic shock syndrome, 47-50; training programs of, 52, 158-59; and USAID, 75, 153; venereal disease program of, 24, 113; and Vietnamese refugees, 99-100; Violence Epidemiology Branch of, 196; and WHO, 93, 154, 159-60, 161; workforce of, 23, 24, 31, 112-14

Central Intelligence Agency (CIA), 88
Champion, Hale, 101
China, 22
chloride, 45-46
cholera, 19, 118-19
Cleere, Roy, 41-42
Cleveland, Harland, 77
Clinton, Bill, 178
Close, William, 12-13
Cochi, Steve, 136
Comprehensive Action in a Smallpox Emergency (CASE), 95-96
Confucius, 108
Congo, Democratic Republic of, 12-14
congressional hearings, 48, 170-73, 245-46; on Legionnaires' disease, 64-66; and Obey, 173-75

Conrad, Connie, 53, 246
Conrad, Lyle, 8, 53, 86, 246
contraception, 217, 220, 221, 229
Cook, Philip, 199
Cooper, Ted, 171
Corbett, Jim, *Man-eaters of Kumaon,* 35, 37
Cordero, Jose, 43-45
Cousins, Norman, 58
Craven, Bob, 62
Crick, Francis H., 26
Curran, Jim, 27, 192, *193*; and AIDS crisis, 210, 211, 216-17, 251
Cutter Laboratories, 117, 134
cyclone syndrome, 90-91

Dahomey (Benin), 75-76
Dan, Bruce, 47-48
Darwin, Charles, 226
Davenport, Joan, 250
Deer, Brian, 145, 146
de Leeuw, Evelyne, 189-90
Denver, CO, 34-36
Department of Defense, 3
Department of Health and Human Services (HHS), 77-78, 233; and injury safety, 197, 198, 199; secretaries of, 201-5
diabetes, 147, 169, 204
Dickey, Jay, 199, 229
Diesh, P., 244
Dingell, John, 176, 177
diphtheria-tetanus-pertussis (DTP) vaccine, 202-3
disability-adjusted life years (DALYs), 169
disaster relief: for Bangladesh cyclone, 90-91; need for centralization in, 92; for Nigerian famine, 80-82; use of surveillance in, 82-85, 91-92, 118
Dole, Bob, 198-99
Donne, John, 107
Dowdle, Walter, 67, 111-12, 113, 248
Downs, Wilbur, 8
Drucker, Peter, 113
Duesberg, Peter, 213-14
Dutta, Mahendra, 244

Ebola, 10-17, 27, 154, 246-47; containment of, 17; history of, 10-11; international response to, 13-14, 78, 92, 237; virus causing, 13-14
Eddins, Don, 91, 249
Eelkema, Robert, 51

Ehrlich, Paul, 157
Einstein, Albert, 26, 109
Eisenhower, Dwight D., 25, 132
Emerging Infectious Diseases, 112
Emory University, 155, 246, 250; and CDC, 24-25, 27
Enders, John, 129-30, 131
Epidemic Intelligence Service (EIS): annual conferences of, 6-7, 31-33, 36, 86; as informal network, 42; investigations by, 43-46, 47-50, 62-68, 134, 150, 180-85; Langmuir as founder of, 6, 21, 22-23, 30; recruitment of officers for, 31; training program of, 32-34, 43
epidemiology, 29-30, 116, 214-15; CDC emphasis on, 22, 28, 107; history of, 19-21
equal employment opportunities, 114-16
errors of omission, 148-49
Euripides, 108
evolution, 105, 226

famine: in Leningrad, 82, 165-66; in Netherlands, 82, 84; in Nigeria, 79-87, *87*; problems of providing food in, 83-84; public health approach to, 86; surveillance systems for, 118
Fansidar, 163-64
Farr, William, 118-19
fatalism, 231-32
Federal Bureau of Investigation (FBI), 1-2
Feynman, Richard, 109
Field Epidemiology Training Program (FETP), 158-59
Finkle, Jack, 176
Finlay, Carlos, 128
First Do No Harm, 148
Food and Drug Administration (FDA), 45, 150, 163, 171, 182, 184, 185, 214
Ford, Gerald, 59
Foster, Stan, 8, 244
Frame, John, 8
Framingham Study, 22
Francis, Don, 13, 247
Francis, Thomas, 38, 130, 132, 133, 250
Franklin, Benjamin, 109, 172
Fraser, David, 62, 65, 66, 67, 247
Fredrickson, Don, 104
Frieden, Thomas, 16
Friendly, Fred, 132
Frost, Wade Hampton, 21, 128
Fulginiti, Vince, 39

Gallo, Robert, 215-16
Gates, Bill, Jr., 222-23, 251
Gates, Bill, Sr., 223, 251
Gayle, Helene, 223
Gelfand, Henry, 70, 74
genetics, 26, 105-6
Gilmartin, Ray, 221
Giordano, Joe, 164
Glass, Roger, 164
Global Alliance for Vaccines and Immunization (GAVI), 143
global warming, 166, 200, 225
Godal, Tore, 143
Google, 119
Gordon, Alexander, *Treatise on the Epidemic of Puerperal Fever,* 20
Gottsdanker, Josephine, 133
Graham, Bob, 171, 246
Grant, Jim, 141, 142, 200, 207
Grasset, Nicole, 245
Guinan, Mary, 251
Guinea, 14, 16
Guinea worm, 219, 249
gun safety, 198-99, 229

Haagen, Eugen, 129
Haley, Mrs. Robert, 48
Hardy, George, 176
Harris, Patricia, 203-4
Harvard School of Public Health, 52-53
Harvard University, 224
Hatch, Orrin, 171-72
Hatfield, Mark, 167, 171, 177-78, 245
health risk appraisal programs, 5-6
Heckler, Margaret, 205, 216, 218
Henderson, D. A., 74, 153, 154
Henderson, Rafe, 91, 125, 141, 154, 159; portrayal of, 81, 249
Henderson-Eddins method, 91
hepatitis, 38, 39, 211; vaccine for, 140
Hesburgh, Theodore, 166
Heymann, David, 62
Hicks, Jim, 74, 81
Hill, Lister, 133
Hilleman, Maurice, 139-40
Hinman, Alan, 136, 250
Hirabayashi, Gordon, 55-57, *57*
Hirabayashi, Jim, 56, 57
Hirabayashi v. the United States, 56
Hobby, Oveta Culp, 132-33
Holmes, Oliver Wendell, Sr., 20

homosexuality, 210, 211, 219
Hong Kong flu, 140
Hongzhi, Emperor, 231
Hope for African Children Initiative (HACI), 223
Hopkins, Don, 77, 155, 249
Horowitz, Larry, 89-90
Hospice (AIDS program), 223
hospital infections, 151-52
Houston, Charles, 36-37, 242
human papillomavirus (HPV) vaccine, 138
Hunter, John, 20

Imhotep, 108
immigrants and refugees, 98-100
immunization. *See* vaccines and immunizations
India: AIDS in, 218; smallpox eradication efforts in, 36-38, 96-97
influenza: and Reye syndrome, 181-86; surveillance system for, 117, 119; vaccines for, 111-12, 113, 138, 140; virus, 7, 58, 59, 63, 101, 113, 130, 248, 250. *See also* swine flu
injury control, 195-99, 247
Injury in America: A Continuing Public Health Problem, 197
Institute of Medicine (IOM), 185, 197
insurance companies, 59-60
International AIDS Vaccine Institute (IAVI), 218
International Committee of the Red Cross (ICRC), 79-80, 88
Isocrates, 188

Jackson, Maynard, 207
Jaffe, Harold, 210
Japanese American internment, 56
Japanese B encephalitis, 140
Jenner, Edward, 20, 127, 139
jet injectors, 39-40, *41*
John, Jacob, 244
Johns Hopkins University, 21
Johnson, George, 180
Johnson, Karl, 11, 246
Johnson, Lyndon, 100, 133
Journal of the American Medical Association (JAMA), 106, 119-20, 206

Kaiser, Robert, 153
Kempe, C. Henry, 39

Kennedy, Edward, 48, 89-90, 171, 245
Kennedy, John F., 38
Kew, Olen, 112-13, 249-50
Keys, Ancel, 81-82
King, Martin Luther, Jr., 114
King-Anderson bill, 168
Kingma, Stuart, 2-3, 90, 243-44
Kissinger, Henry, 89-90
Kohlstedt, Shirley and Jim, 241
Koop, C. Everett, 200-201, 221, 245
Korean hemorrhagic fever, 22

Lagos, Nigeria, 81, 193-94
Lancet, 144, 145, 179-80
Lane, Mike, 74, 94, 248-49
Langmuir, Alexander, 43, 86, 107; and Cutter incident, 133-34; and founding of EIS, 6, 21, 22-23, 30; global interests of, 153; and polio vaccine, 34, 126; portrayal of, 6n, 242
Laskin, Carol, 45
Lassa fever, 7-10, 179
Last Chance Diet, The, 150
lead poisoning, 203-4
League of the Red Cross, 79
Lee, Phil, 162, 178
Legionnaires' disease, 60-68, 179, 210, 247; CDC investigation of, 62-68; CDC resolution of, 66-68; Congress on, 64-66, 68; *Legionella* bacterium causing, 60-61, 158; as public health emergency, 60-62
Lehman, Bill, 171, 197, 198, 245-46
Leibler, Seth, 95, 110, 249
Leibowitch, Jacques, 215
Leningrad famine, 82, 165-66
leprosy, 100, 112, 248
Lewis, John, 114, 207
Liberia, 14, 16, 74
Lichfield, Paul, 71
life expectancy, 32, 152, 187-88, 205
liquid protein diets, 150-51
Lokela, Mabalo, 10, 11
Lott, Trent, 198-99
Louis, Pierre Charles Alexandre, 20
Lucas, Adetokunbo, 193-94, 243
Lukwiya, Matthew, 14-16, *15*
Lundberg, George, 119-20
Lutheran Church-Missouri Synod (LCMS), 53-55
Lythcott, George, 81, 175, 249

Macdonald, Guy, 222
Mahler, Halfdan, 142, 207
malaria, 21, 99, 153; prophylaxis for, 69-70,
    163; surveillance systems for, 117, 133
Malaria Control Program, 21, 22, 113
Mali, 16
Manley, Michael, 231
Mann, Jonathan, 154
marketplace, 149, 167-68, 169, 230
Mason, Jim, 237
maternal mortality, 19
Mather, Anne, 251
Matthews, Gene, 248
Mays, Benjamin, 114
Mbeki, Thabo, 213-14
McCormick, Joseph, 9-10, 11, 247
McDade, Joseph, 66-67, 68, 112, 247-48
McGill, Ralph, 114
McGinnis, J. Michael, 106, 125
McNamara, Robert, 141
measles: CDC Africa program around, 47,
    75-77, 83; deaths from, 47, 75, 83, 187;
    immunization for, 38-39, 136-38
Measles, mumps, and rubella (MMR)
    vaccine, 129, 140; and autism, 144, 145
Mectizan, 221
Meiklejohn, Gordon, 35-36
Memphis, TN, 43-44, 128
meningitis, 81, 83, 138
Merck, 140, 221-22, 223, 224
Merieux, Charles, 139
Merson, Mike, 154
Millar, J. Donald, 30, 80, 110; and NIOSH,
    176, 178; portrayal of, 135-36, 244; and
    Smallpox Eradication Program, 74, 93, 96,
    136
Millennium Development Goals (MDGs), 125
Miller, Frank, 156
Mills, William Mervin "Billy," 122-23
Mobutu Sese Seko, 12, 13
"Mohan Singh," 189-91
Mollahan, Cecil, 35
Montagnier, Luc, 215-16
Morbidity and Mortality Weekly Report
    (MMWR), 67-68, 100, 151, 163-64, 248, 251;
    about, 119-20; on AIDS, 209, 211, 214-15;
    on Reye syndrome, 180, 181-82, 183-86
Morgan, Graeme, 179-80
Morris, Leo, 93
mortality statistics, 106, 110, 165-66
Mosley, Henry, 90-91

Mountin, Joseph, 22, 25
Murphy, John M., 64-65, 68, 171
Murrow, Edward R., 132
Museveni, Yoweri, 218

Nader, Ralph, 140
Najjar, Ed, 155
Nakajima, Hiroshi, 142
Nakano, Jim, 96
Natcher, William, 171
National Center for Injury Prevention and
    Control, 199
National Foundation for Infantile Paralysis,
    131
National Institute for Occupational Safety
    and Health (NIOSH), 175-78
National Institutes of Health (NIH), 104,
    176-78, 215-16, 219, 234
National Rifle Association (NRA), 198, 229
Native Americans, 122-23
Neff, John, 94
Neo Mull Soy, 44-45
Netherlands famine, 82, 84
Neva, Frank, 52, 53, 242
nicotine addiction, 143-44
Nigeria, 53-55, 69-70, 73-74; civil war in,
    56-57, 72, 73, 79; and Ebola, 16-17; famine
    and relief efforts in, 80-90, 162; and
    malaria, 69-70; and smallpox, 70-73; tribal
    hostilities in, 193-94
Nixon, Richard, 89
Nkinsi, Luke, 224
Noguchi, Hideyo, 128-29
North Atlantic Treaty Organization (NATO),
    92

Obey, David, 173, 174-75, 177-78
Ochelebe, Lawrence Atutu, 70-71, 80-81
Offit, Paul, 133
Ogden, Hod, 31, 189-91, 192
Orenstein, Walter, 136, 250

Panama Canal, 128
Pan American Health Organization, 138, 160
Paris, Nancy, 219
partnerships, 119-20
Pasteur, Louis, 139
Pasteur Institute, 215-17
Patek, A. J., 213
Paul, Ron, 168
Peace Corps, 36-37

Pediatrics, 181, 184
Percy, Charles, 150-51
PERT chart, 95
Phipps, James, 20
Pilot, Lynn, 45
Pinneo, Lily Lyman, 7-8, 9
Piot, Peter, 11, 12, 247
Plantation News, 114
pneumonia, 61, 62, 67-68, 99, 164, 247; and
    AIDS, 209, 211; vaccine for, 138
polio, 133, 249; declining incidence of, 131,
    134; last outbreak of, 134-35; terrorists'
    targeting of vaccinators against, 147
polio vaccine: and Cutter incident, 133-34;
    federal responsibility for providing, 120,
    132-33; field test for, 130, 132, 133, 250;
    risks of, 34-36, 152; Sabin oral vaccine,
    34, 59, 134, 152; Salk development of,
    38, 52, 129-32; surveillance system
    for, 117
politics: and NIOSH, 175-78; and politicians,
    17, 162-78; and public health, 48, 162, 166;
    science pushed aside by, 160, 213-14; and
    USAID, 77-78
polling, 91, 249
Polybius, 108, 233
Pontiac, MI, 66
Pool, Judith, 213
poverty, 230-31
President's Emergency Plan for AIDS Relief
    (PEPFAR), 161, 221
prevention, 149; and public health, 32,
    167-68, 169
public health: and appropriate response, 118,
    124-25; and behavior change, 46, 225; as
    CDC mission, 30, 104, 105-6, 120-21;
    clinical medicine difference with, 50, 152;
    first school of, 21; funding of, 167-69;
    historical wisdom on, 108-10; immuniza-
    tion as foundation of, 126, 143-44, 147, 235;
    and marketplace, 149, 167-68, 169, 230; and
    politics, 48, 162, 166; and poverty, 230-31;
    and prevention, 32, 167-68, 169; require-
    ments for programs of, 18, 46; science as
    bedrock of, 28, 200, 204; single-payer
    system for, 149, 169, 230; and violence, 106,
    195, 198
Public Health Service, 24, 114, 116; budget of,
    233; CDC as delivery arm of, 104;
    objectives of, 125
Public Law 96-359, 45

QUAC stick, 85
Quadros, Ciro de, 93

Rabelais, 109
Ramalingaswami, Vulimiri, 218
Ravenholt, Rei, 30, 31, 106, 242
Reagan, Ronald, 204, 205, 234
Red Book Committee, 110
Red Cross. *See* International Committee of
    the Red Cross
Reed, Walter, 128
refugee camps, 84-85, 162-66
Reingold, Art, 47-48
Reinstein, Cecil, 5-6
religious beliefs, 98, 135, 221, 226-27, 229
Rely tampons, 49-50
Reye, Douglas, 179-80
Reye syndrome, 179-86; about, 179-80; and
    CDC, 180-85; and salicylates, 180-86;
    solution to problem of, 185-86; studies of,
    180, 181, 184-86
rich and poor, 30-31
Richmond, Julius, 125, 158, 176, 203;
    portrayal of, 245; and refugee camps, 162,
    163, 164
risk: calculating, 49-50; and hospital
    infections, 152; and vaccines, 94-95, 135,
    152
Robbins, Fred, 129-30, 131
Robbins, Tony, 176
Roberto, Ron, 40
Robinson, Roslyn "Robbie," 67
Rockefeller Foundation, 128-29, 141, 217,
    218
Rocky Mountain spotted fever, 4-5
Rogers, Paul, 171, 245
Rollin, Pierre, 16
Roman, Juan, 8
Roosevelt, Franklin, 131
Rosenberg, Mark, 142, 196, 197, 198, 199, 247
Ross, Sir Ronald, 128
Rwanda genocide, 166

Sabin, Albert, 59. *See also* polio vaccine
Salk, Jonas, 59, 141; and polio vaccine, 38,
    130, 131-32, 138, 139, 141
Salote, Queen, 40
Sanders, Robert, 196
Satcher, David, 178
Saunders, Dame Cicely, 223
Schnitker, Paul, 86

Schweiker, Richard, 159, 171, 183; and CDC budget, 233, 235, 236-37; portrayal of, 204-5, 245

Schweitzer, Albert, 109; *Out of My Life and Thought,* 51

security practices, 4-6

Selecky, Mary, 200

Semmelweiss, Ignaz, 19

Sencer, David, 88, 89, 99, *101*, 137, 156; and equal employment opportunities, 114, 115-16; and global health issues, 90-91, 153, 154; humor by, 188-89, 191; and Legionnaires' disease, 65, 67-68; portrayal of, 243; and swine flu epidemic, 59, 101-2, 171

Senegal, 14, 16

sensitivity sessions, 114

Serfling, Robert E., 91

Shands, Kathy, 47-48

Sharma, M. I. D., 244

Sharrar, Bob, 62

Shaw, George Bernard, 188

Shepard, Charles, 67-68, 112, 248

Sherman, Ida L., 91

Sierra Leone, 14, 16, 77, 247, 249

Simon, Paul, 171, 245

single-payer system, 149, 169, 230

slavery, 108, 227, 231

smallpox: CASE program for, 95-96; in eastern Nigeria, 70-73; evolution of virus causing, 76; immunization against, in Africa, 71-73, 74-75, 76; India's eradication efforts against, 5, 36, 96-97; as seasonal disease, 76; surveillance/containment strategy toward, 72, 74-76, 83, 97; West Africa elimination of, 5, 77-78

Smallpox Eradication Program, 13, 70, 83, 91, 93, 153, 154

smallpox vaccine: Jenner efforts toward, 20, 127, 139; risks of, 94-95, 248-49

Snow, John, 19, 118-19

Sommer, Al, 90-91

South Africa, 213-14

Soviet Union, 157-58, 205-6

Spector, Arlen, 199

speeches, 121-23

Staphylococcus infections, 19, 32

Starko, Karen, 180, 181

State Department, 77, 86-88, 158, 205-6

Steffens, Lincoln, 172

Stewart, William H. "Bill," *41*

Stockman, David, 236

Stokes, Adrian, 128

Stonesifer, Patty, 251

Strunk, Bill, 241-42

Stuart, Johannes, 24

Sudan, 10, 13-14, 207, 247

Summit for Children, 142-43

surveillance and containment approach, 71, 72, 74-77, 97

surveillance systems, 49-50, 71, 133, 186; for abortion, 200-201, 245; for famine, 82-90, 118; history of, 117, 118-19; hospitals with, 151-52; and relief efforts, 82-85, 91-92, 118

swine flu: CDC response to, 58-60; criticisms of CDC around, 49, 101, 202; immunization program for, 61-62, 101

Syntex Corporation, 44-45

Task Force for Child Survival, 141-42, 157, 217, 221

Task Force for Global Health, 142-43, 247

Taylor, F. H. L., 213

Tejada de Rivero, David, 157

Tennessee Child Passenger Safety Law, 196

tetanus vaccine, 130

Thacker, Steve, 62

Thailand, 159; refugee camps in, 162-66

Theiler, Max, 129

Thompson, David, 71, 248

Thompson, Joan, 71

Thurman, Sandy, 219

tobacco, 32, 143-44, 146, 168, 171, 175, 187-88, 203, 227-28

Tonga, 39-40

Tort Claim Act, 61-62

toxic shock syndrome (TSS), 7, 47-50

Troup, Jeanette, 9, 246

tuberculosis, 30, 81, 99, 100, 121, 164

Twain, Mark, 166, 205

typhoid fever, 35, 99

UNICEF, 141, 142, 154, 157

United Nations Development Programme (UNDP), 141, 154

United States Agency for International Development (USAID), 75, 77-78, 141, 153, 159

vaccines and immunizations: and AIDS, 220; anticancer, 138, 147; and autism, 144-46; BCG, 53; concept behind, 126, 129; DTP,

vaccines and immunizations (*cont.*)
202-3; education around, 143-44, 147;
federal regulation of, 134; as foundation of
public health, 126, 143-44, 147, 235; future
of, 147; hepatitis, 140; history of, 127-29,
138-39; HPV, 138; influenza, 111-12, 113,
138, 140; jet injectors for, 39-40, *41*; for
measles, 38-39, 136-38; MMR, 129, 140,
144, 145; national immunization program,
135-36; polio, 35-36, 38, 52, 117, 120,
129-34, 135-36, 152, 250; and risks, 94-95,
135, 152, 248-49; rubella, 138; smallpox, 20,
72-73, 74-75, 76, 94-95, 127, 139, 248-49; as
social contract, 132-33; Swine Flu
Program, 59-60; and Task Force for Child
Survival, 141-42; tetanus, 130; and
thimerosal, 144; yellow fever, 127-28
Vagelos, Roy, 140, 221
Venediktov, Dimitri, 157-58
Vietnamese refugees, 99-100
Villa International, 155
violence, 106, 195, 196, 198
Vonnegut, Kurt, 24, 227

Wakefield, Andrew, 144, 145-46
Walters, Carol, 1, 178, 250

Watson, Bill, 113, 158, 166, 176, 178, 243;
portrayal of, 24
Watson, James, *The Double Helix,* 26
Waxman, Henry, 150, 171, 245
Wecht, Cyril, 64
Weiss, Ted, 172-73
Weller, Tom, 51-53, 129-30, 131, 155, 242
Western, Karl, 86, 89
White, Mike, 11
Wiesner, Paul, 210, 250
women: in Africa, 217; in EIS, 241; in
medical school, 241; as voters, 226-27
Woodruff, Robert, 25
World Bank, 141, 154, 169
World Health Organization (WHO), 89, 129,
141, 153; and CDC, 93, 153, 154, 159-60, 161;
and Ebola epidemic, 11-17; and UNICEF,
157

yellow fever, 127-29
Young, Andrew, 114, 207
Young, William, 129

Zaire, 10-13, 247
Zhdanov, Viktor Mikhailovich, 158
Zimbardo, Philip, 170-71